MCAT®

Biochemistry Review

2nd Edition

The Staff of The Princeton Review

Penguin
Random
House

The Princeton Review
110 E. 42nd Street, 7th Floor
New York, NY 10017

Published in the United States by Penguin Random House
LLC, New York, and in Canada by Random House of Canada,
a division of Penguin Random House Ltd., Toronto.

Terms of Service: The Princeton Review Online Companion
Tools ("Student Tools") for retail books are available for only
the two most recent editions of that book. Student Tools
may be activated only once per eligible book purchased
for a total of 24 months of access. Activation of Student
Tools more than once per book is in direct violation of these
Terms of Service and may result in discontinuation of
access to Student Tools Services.

ISBN: 978-0-593-51621-8
ISSN: 2380-7741

MCAT is a registered trademark of the Association of
American Medical Colleges.

The Princeton Review is not affiliated with Princeton
University.

The material in this book is up-to-date at the time of pub-
lication. However, changes may have been instituted by the
testing body in the test after this book was published.

If there are any important late-breaking developments,
changes, or corrections to the materials in this book, we
will post that information online in the Student Tools.
Register your book and check your Student Tools to see if
there are any updates posted there.

Every attempt has been made to obtain permission to
reproduce material protected by copyright. Where
omissions may have occurred the editors will be happy
to acknowledge this in future printings.

Permission has been granted to reprint portions of the
following

From The New England Journal of Medicine, Kevin Fitzgerald,
Suellen White, Anna Borodovsky, et al, A Highly Durable RNAi
Therapeutic Inhibitor of PCSK9, Volume 376, Copyright © 2017
Massachusetts Medical Society. Reprinted with permission from
Massachusetts Medical Society.

Reprinted by permission from Springer Nature Customer Service
Centre GmbH: Springer Nature, Molecular and Cellular Biochemistry, Nerolidol, a sesquiterpene, attenuates oxidative stress and
inflammation in acetic acid-induced colitis in rats, Salim M. A.
Bastaki et al, © 2021

The Princeton Review Publishing Team
Rob Franek, Editor-in-Chief
David Soto, Senior Director, Data Operations
Stephen Koch, Senior Manager, Data Operations
Deborah Weber, Director of Production
Jason Ullmeyer, Production Design Manager
Jennifer Chapman, Senior Production Artist
Selena Coppock, Director of Editorial
Aaron Riccio, Senior Editor
Meave Shelton, Senior Editor
Chris Chimera, Editor
Orion McBean, Editor
Patricia Murphy, Editor
Laura Rose, Editor
Alexa Schmitt Bugler, Editorial Assistant

Random House Publishing Team
Tom Russell, VP, Publisher
Alison Stoltzfus, Senior Director, Publishing
Brett Wright, Senior Editor
Emily Hoffman, Assistant Managing Editor
Ellen Reed, Production Manager
Suzanne Lee, Designer
Eugenia Lo, Publishing Assistant

For customer service, please contact
editorialsupport@review.com,
and be sure to include:

- full title of the book

- ISBN

- page number

Editor: Chris Chimera
Production Editors: Kathy Carter and Lyssa Mandel
Production Artist: Jason Ullmeyer

Manufactured in China.

10 9 8 7 6 5 4 3 2 1

2nd Edition

CONTRIBUTORS

Daniel J. Pallin, M.D.
    Senior Author
Judene Wright, M.S., M.A.Ed.
    Senior Author

TPR MCAT Biology and Biochemistry Development Team:

Jessica Adams, Ph.D.

Britney McMurren, B.H.Sc., M.Sc.

Judene Wright, M.S., M.A.Ed., Senior Editor, Lead Developer

Sarah Woodruff, B.S., B.A.

Edited for Production by:

Judene Wright, M.S., M.A.Ed.
    National Content Director, MCAT Program, The Princeton Review

The TPR MCAT Biology and Biochemistry Team and Judene would like to thank the following people for their contributions to this book:

Kashif Anwar, M.D., M.M.S., John Bahling, M.D., Kristen Brunson, Ph.D., Phil Carpenter, Ph.D., Khawar Chaudry, B.S., Nita Chauhan, H.BSc, MSc, Dan Cho, M.P.H., Glenn E. Croston, Ph.D., Nathan Deal, M.D., Ian Denham, B.Sc., B.Ed., Joshua Dilworth, M.D., Ph.D., Annie Dude, Rob Fong, M.D., Ph.D., Chris Fortenbach, B.S., Kirsten Frank, Ph.D., Isabel L. Jackson, B.S., Erik Kildebeck, George Kyriazis, Ph.D., Ben Lee, Heather Liwanag, Ph.D., Travis MacKoy, B.S., Joey Mancuso, M.S., D.O., Evan Martow, BMSc, Brian Mikolasko, M.D., M.BA, Abhisehk Mohapatra, B.A., Christopher Moriates, M.D., Stephen L. Nelson, Jr., Ph.D., Rupal Patel, B.S., Mary Qiu, Ina C. Roy, M.D., Jayson Sack, M.D., M.S., Will Sanderson, Jeanine Seitz-Partridge, M.S., Oktay Shuminov, B.S., Andrew D. Snyder, M.D., Preston Swirnoff, Ph.D., M.S.,Jenkang Tao, B.S., B.A., Rhead Uddin, Jia Wang.

PERIODIC TABLE OF THE ELEMENTS

1																	18
1 **H** 1.0	2											13	14	15	16	17	2 **He** 4.0
3 **Li** 6.9	4 **Be** 9.0											5 **B** 10.8	6 **C** 12.0	7 **N** 14.0	8 **O** 16.0	9 **F** 19.0	10 **Ne** 20.2
11 **Na** 23.0	12 **Mg** 24.3	3	4	5	6	7	8	9	10	11	12	13 **Al** 27.0	14 **Si** 28.1	15 **P** 31.0	16 **S** 32.1	17 **Cl** 35.5	18 **Ar** 39.9
19 **K** 39.1	20 **Ca** 40.1	21 **Sc** 45.0	22 **Ti** 47.9	23 **V** 50.9	24 **Cr** 52.0	25 **Mn** 54.9	26 **Fe** 55.8	27 **Co** 58.9	28 **Ni** 58.7	29 **Cu** 63.5	30 **Zn** 65.4	31 **Ga** 69.7	32 **Ge** 72.6	33 **As** 74.9	34 **Se** 79.0	35 **Br** 79.9	36 **Kr** 83.8
37 **Rb** 85.5	38 **Sr** 87.6	39 **Y** 88.9	40 **Zr** 91.2	41 **Nb** 92.9	42 **Mo** 95.9	43 **Tc** (98)	44 **Ru** 101.1	45 **Rh** 102.9	46 **Pd** 106.4	47 **Ag** 107.9	48 **Cd** 112.4	49 **In** 114.8	50 **Sn** 118.7	51 **Sb** 121.8	52 **Te** 127.6	53 **I** 126.9	54 **Xe** 131.3
55 **Cs** 132.9	56 **Ba** 137.3	57 *****La** 138.9	72 **Hf** 178.5	73 **Ta** 180.9	74 **W** 183.9	75 **Re** 186.2	76 **Os** 190.2	77 **Ir** 192.2	78 **Pt** 195.1	79 **Au** 197.0	80 **Hg** 200.6	81 **Tl** 204.4	82 **Pb** 207.2	83 **Bi** 209.0	84 **Po** (209)	85 **At** (210)	86 **Rn** (222)
87 **Fr** (223)	88 **Ra** (226)	89 **†Ac** (227)	104 **Rf** (267)	105 **Db** (268)	106 **Sg** (271)	107 **Bh** (270)	108 **Hs** (269)	109 **Mt** (278)	110 **Ds** (281)	111 **Rg** (282)	112 **Cn** (285)	113 **Nh** (286)	114 **Fl** (289)	115 **Mc** (289)	116 **Lv** (293)	117 **Ts** (294)	118 **Og** (294)

*Lanthanoids	58 **Ce** 140.1	59 **Pr** 140.9	60 **Nd** 144.2	61 **Pm** (145)	62 **Sm** 150.4	63 **Eu** 152.0	64 **Gd** 157.3	65 **Tb** 158.9	66 **Dy** 162.5	67 **Ho** 164.9	68 **Er** 167.3	69 **Tm** 168.9	70 **Yb** 173.0	71 **Lu** 175.0
†Actinoids	90 **Th** 232.0	91 **Pa** (231)	92 **U** 238.0	93 **Np** (237)	94 **Pu** (244)	95 **Am** (243)	96 **Cm** (247)	97 **Bk** (247)	98 **Cf** (251)	99 **Es** (252)	100 **Fm** (257)	101 **Md** (258)	102 **No** (259)	103 **Lr** (266)

CONTENTS

Get More (Free) Content
at **PrincetonReview.com/prep**

As easy as **1·2·3**

1 Go to PrincetonReview.com/prep or scan the **QR code** and enter the following ISBN for your book:
9780593516218

2 Answer a few simple questions to set up an exclusive Princeton Review account. *(If you already have one, you can just log in.)*

3 Enjoy access to your **FREE** content!

Once you've registered, you can...

- Take **3** full-length practice MCAT exams

- Find useful information about taking the MCAT and applying to medical school

- Check to see if there have been any corrections or updates to this edition

- Get our take on any recent or pending updates to the MCAT

Need to report a potential **content** issue?

Contact **EditorialSupport@review.com** and include:

- full title of the book
- ISBN
- page number

Need to report a **technical** issue?

Contact **TPRStudentTech@review.com** and provide:

- your full name
- email address used to register the book
- full book title and ISBN
- Operating system (Mac/PC) and browser (Chrome, Firefox, Safari, etc.)

Chapter 1
MCAT Basics

SO YOU WANT TO BE A DOCTOR

So...you want to be a doctor. If you're like most premeds, you've wanted to be a doctor since you were pretty young. When people asked you what you wanted to be when you grew up, you always answered "a doctor." You had toy medical kits, bandaged up your dog or cat, and played "hospital." You probably read your parents' home medical guides for fun.

When you got to high school you took the honors and AP classes. You studied hard, got straight A's (or at least really good grades!), and participated in extracurricular activities so you could get into a good college. And you succeeded!

At college you knew exactly what to do. You took your classes seriously, studied hard, and got a great GPA. You talked to your professors and hung out at office hours to get good letters of recommendation. You were a member of the premed society on campus, volunteered at hospitals, and shadowed doctors. All that's left to do now is get a good MCAT score.

Just the MCAT.

Just the most confidence-shattering, most demoralizing, longest, most brutal entrance exam for any graduate program. At about 7.5 hours (including breaks), the MCAT tops the list...even the closest runners up, the LSAT and GMAT, are only about 4 hours long. The MCAT tests significant science content knowledge along with the ability to think quickly, reason logically, and read comprehensively, all under the pressure of a timed exam.

The path to a good MCAT score is not as easy to see as the path to a good GPA or the path to a good letter of recommendation. The MCAT is less about what you know, and more about how to apply what you know...and how to apply it quickly to new situations. Because the path might not be so clear, you might be worried. That's why you picked up this book.

We promise to demystify the MCAT for you, with clear descriptions of the different sections, how the test is scored, and what the test experience is like. We will help you understand general test-taking techniques as well as provide you with specific techniques for each section. We will review the science content you need to know as well as give you strategies for the Critical Analysis and Reasoning Skills (CARS) section. We'll show you the path to a good MCAT score and help you walk the path.

After all...you want to be a doctor. And we want you to succeed.

WHAT IS THE MCAT...REALLY?

Most test-takers approach the MCAT as though it were a typical college science test, one in which facts and knowledge simply need to be regurgitated in order to do well. They study for the MCAT the same way they did for their college tests, by memorizing facts and details, formulas and equations. And when they get to the MCAT, they are surprised...and disappointed.

It's a myth that the MCAT is purely a content-knowledge test. If medical-school admission committees want to see what you know, all they have to do is look at your transcripts. What they really want to see is how you think, especially under pressure. That's what your MCAT score will tell them.

The MCAT is really a test of your ability to apply basic knowledge to different, possibly new, situations. It's a test of your ability to reason out and evaluate arguments. Do you still need to know your science content? Absolutely. But not at the level that most test-takers think they need to know it. Furthermore, your science knowledge won't help you on the Critical Analysis and Reasoning Skills (CARS) section. So how do you study for a test like this?

You study for the science sections by reviewing the basics and then applying them to MCAT practice questions. You study for the CARS section by learning how to adapt your existing reading and analytical skills to the nature of the test (more information about the CARS section can be found in *MCAT Critical Analysis and Reasoning Skills Review*).

The book you are holding will review all the relevant MCAT Biochemistry content you will need for the test and a little bit more. It includes hundreds of questions designed to make you think about the material in a deeper way, along with full explanations to clarify the logical thought process needed to get to the answer. It also comes with access to three full-length online practice exams to further hone your skills. For more information on accessing those online exams, please refer to the "Get More (Free) Content" spread on page viii.

MCAT NUTS AND BOLTS

Overview

The MCAT is a computer-based test (CBT) that is *not* adaptive. Adaptive tests base your next question on whether or not you've answered the current question correctly. The MCAT is *linear*, or *fixed-form*, meaning that the questions are in a predetermined order and do not change based on your answers. However, there are many versions of the test, so that on a given test day, different people will see different versions. The following table highlights the features of the MCAT exam.

Registration	Online via www.aamc.org. Begins as early as six months prior to test date; available up until week of test (subject to seat availability).
Testing Centers	Administered at small, secure, climate-controlled computer testing rooms.
Security	Photo ID with signature, electronic fingerprint, electronic signature verification, assigned seat.
Proctoring	None. Test administrator checks examinee in and assigns seat at computer. All testing instructions are given on the computer.
Frequency of Test	Many times per year distributed over January, April, May, June, July, August, and September.
Format	Exclusively computer-based. NOT an adaptive test.
Length of Test Day	7.5 hours
Breaks	Optional 10-minute breaks between sections, with a 30-minute break for lunch.
Section Names	1. Chemical and Physical Foundations of Biological Systems (Chem/Phys) 2. Critical Analysis and Reasoning Skills (CARS) 3. Biological and Biochemical Foundations of Living Systems (Bio/Biochem) 4. Psychological, Social, and Biological Foundations of Behavior (Psych/Soc)
Number of Questions and Timing	59 Chem/Phys questions, 95 minutes 53 CARS questions, 90 minutes 59 Bio/Biochem questions, 95 minutes 59 Psych/Soc questions, 95 minutes
Scoring	Test is scaled. Several forms per administration.
Allowed/ Not allowed	No timers/watches. Noise reduction headphones available. Noteboard booklet and wet-erase marker given at start of test and taken at end of test. Locker or secure area provided for personal items.
Results: Timing and Delivery	Approximately 30 days. Electronic scores only, available online through AAMC login. Examinees can print official score reports.
Maximum Number of Retakes	The test can be taken a maximum of three times in one year, four times over two years, and seven times over the lifetime of the examinee. An examinee can be registered for only one date at a time.

Registration

Registration for the exam is completed online at www.aamc.org/students/applying/mcat/reserving. The AAMC opens registration for a given test date at least two months in advance of the date, often earlier. It's a good idea to register well in advance of your desired test date to make sure that you get a seat.

Sections

There are four sections on the MCAT exam: Chemical and Physical Foundations of Biological Systems (Chem/Phys), Critical Analysis and Reasoning Skills (CARS), Biological and Biochemical Foundations of Living Systems (Bio/Biochem), and Psychological, Social, and Biological Foundations of Behavior (Psych/Soc). All sections consist of multiple-choice questions.

Section	Concepts Tested	Number of Questions and Timing
Chemical and Physical Foundations of Biological Systems	Basic concepts in chemistry and physics, including biochemistry, scientific inquiry, reasoning, research and statistics skills.	59 questions in 95 minutes
Critical Analysis and Reasoning Skills	Critical analysis of information drawn from a wide range of social science and humanities disciplines.	53 questions in 90 minutes
Biological and Biochemical Foundations of Living Systems	Basic concepts in biology and biochemistry, scientific inquiry, reasoning, research and statistics skills.	59 questions in 95 minutes
Psychological, Social, and Biological Foundations of Behavior	Basic concepts in psychology, sociology, biology, research methods, and statistics.	59 questions in 95 minutes

Most questions on the MCAT (44 in the science sections, all 53 in the CARS section) are passage-based; the science sections have 10 passages each, and the CARS section has 9. A passage consists of a few paragraphs of information on which several following questions are based. In the science sections, passages often include equations or reactions, tables, graphs, figures, and experiments to analyze. CARS passages come from literature in social sciences, humanities, ethics, philosophy, cultural studies, and population health, and do not test content knowledge in any way.

Some questions in the science sections are freestanding questions (FSQs). These questions are independent of any passage information and appear in four groups of about three to four questions, interspersed throughout the passages. In the science sections, 15 of the question are freestanding, and the remainder are passage-based.

Each section on the MCAT is separated by either a 10-minute break or a 30-minute lunch break. We recommend that you take these breaks.

Section	Time
Test Center Check-In	Variable, can take up to 40 minutes if center is busy.
Tutorial	10 minutes
Chemical and Physical Foundations of Biological Systems	95 minutes
Break (optional)	10 minutes
Critical Analysis and Reasoning Skills	90 minutes
Lunch Break (optional)	30 minutes
Biological and Biochemical Foundations of Living Systems	95 minutes
Break (optional)	10 minutes
Psychological, Social, and Biological Foundations of Behavior	95 minutes
Void Option	5 minutes
Survey (optional)	5 minutes

The survey includes questions about your satisfaction with the overall MCAT experience, including registration, check-in, etc., as well as questions about how you prepared for the test.

Scoring

The MCAT is a scaled exam, meaning that your raw score will be converted into a scaled score that takes into account the difficulty of the questions. There is no guessing penalty. All sections are scored from 118–132, with a total scaled score range of 472–528. Because different versions of the test have varying levels of difficulty, the scale will be different from one exam to the next. Thus, there is no "magic number" of questions to get right in order to get a particular score. Plus, some of the questions on the test are considered "experimental" and do not count toward your score; they are just there to be evaluated for possible future inclusion in a test.

At the end of the test (after you complete the Psychological, Social, and Biological Foundations of Behavior section), you will be asked to choose one of the following two options, "I wish to have my MCAT exam scored" or "I wish to VOID my MCAT exam." You have five minutes to make a decision, and if you do not select one of the options in that time, the test will automatically be scored. If you choose the VOID option, your test will not be scored (you will not now, or ever, receive a numerical score for this test), medical schools will not know you took the test, and no refunds will be granted. You cannot "unvoid" your scores at a later time.

So, what's a good score? The AAMC is centering the scale at 500 (i.e., 500 will be the 50th percentile), and recommends that application committees consider applicants near the center of the range. To be on the safe side, aim for a total score of around 510. Remember that if your GPA is on the low side, you'll need higher MCAT scores to compensate, and if you have a strong GPA, you can get away with lower MCAT scores. But the reality is that your chances of acceptance depend on a lot more than just your MCAT scores. It's a combination of your GPA, your MCAT scores, your undergraduate coursework, letters of recommendation, experience related to the medical field (such as volunteer work or research), extracurricular activities, your personal statement, etc. Medical schools are looking for a complete package, not just good scores and a good GPA.

GENERAL LAYOUT AND TEST-TAKING STRATEGIES

Layout of the Test

In each section of the test, the computer screen is divided vertically, with the passage on the left and the range of questions for that passage indicated above (e.g., "Passage 1 Questions 1–5"). The scroll bar for the passage text appears in the middle of the screen. Each question appears on the right, and you need to click "Next" to move to each subsequent question.

In the science sections, the freestanding questions are found in groups of 3–4, interspersed with the passages. The screen is still divided vertically; on the left is the statement "Questions [X–XX] do not refer to a passage and are independent of each other," and each question appears on the right as described above.

CBT Tools

There are a number of tools available on the test, including highlighting, strike-outs, the Flag for Review button, the Navigation and Review Screen buttons, the Periodic Table button, and of course, the noteboard booklet. All tools are available with both mouse control (buttons to click) or keyboard commands (Alt+ a letter). As everyone has different preferences, you should practice with both types of tools (mouse and keyboard) to see which is more comfortable for you personally. The following is a brief description of each tool.

1) **Highlighting:** This is done in the passage text (including table entries and some equations, but excluding figures and molecular structures), in the question stems, and in the answer choices (including Roman numerals). Select the words you wish to highlight (left-click and drag the cursor across the words), and in the upper left corner click the "Highlight" button to highlight the selected text yellow. Alternatively, press "Alt+H" to highlight the words. Highlighting can be removed by selecting the words again and in the upper left corner clicking the down arrow next to "Highlight." This will expand to show the "Remove Highlight" option; clicking this will remove the highlighting. Removing highlighting via the keyboard is cumbersome and is not recommended.

2) **Strike-outs:** This can be done on the answer choices, including Roman numeral statements, by selecting the text you want to strike out (left-click and drag the cursor across the text) and then clicking the "Strikethrough" button in the upper left corner. Alternatively, press "Alt+S" to strike out the words. The strike-out can be removed by repeating these actions. **Figures or molecular structures cannot be struck out; however, the letter answer choice of those structures can.**

3) **Flag for Review button:** This is available for each question and is found in the upper right corner. This allows you to flag the question as one you would like to review later if time permits. When clicked, the flag icon turns yellow. Click again to remove the flag. Alternatively, press "Alt+F."

4) **Navigation button:** This is found near the bottom of the screen and is available only on your first pass through the section. Clicking this button brings up a navigation table listing all questions and their statuses (unseen, incomplete, complete, flagged for review). You can also press "Alt+N" to bring up the screen. The questions can be sorted by their statuses, and clicking a question number takes you immediately to that question. Once you have reached the end of the section and viewed the Review screen (described below), the Navigation screen is no longer available.

5) **Review Screen button:** This button is found near the bottom of the screen after your first pass through the section. When the button is clicked, it brings up a new screen showing all questions and their statuses (either incomplete, unseen, or flagged for review). Questions that are complete are assigned no additional status. You can then choose one of three options by clicking with the mouse or with keyboard

shortcuts: Review All (Alt+A), Review Incomplete (Alt+I), or Review Flagged (Alt+R); alternatively, you can click a question number to go directly back to that question. You can also end the section from this screen.

6) **Periodic Table button:** Clicking this button will open a periodic table (or press "Alt+T"). Note that the periodic table is large, covering most of the screen. However, this window can be resized to see the questions and a portion of the periodic table at the same time. The table text will not decrease, but scroll bars will appear on the window so you can center the section of the table of interest in the window.

7) **Noteboard Booklet (Scratch Paper):** At the start of the test, you will be given a spiral-bound set of four laminated 8.5"×14" sheets of paper and a wet-erase black marker to use as scratch paper. You can request a clean noteboard booklet at any time during the test; your original booklet will be collected. The noteboard is useful only if it is kept organized; do not give in to the tendency to write on the first available open space! Good organization will be very helpful when/if you wish to review a question. Indicate the passage number, the range of questions for that passage, and a topic in a box near the top of your scratch work, and indicate the question you are working on in a circle to the left of the notes for that question. Draw a line under your scratch work when you change passages to keep the work separate. Do not erase or scribble over any previous work. If you do not think it is correct, draw one line through the work and start again. You may have already done some useful work without realizing it.

General Strategy for the Science Sections

Passages vs. FSQs in the Science Sections: What to Start With

Since the questions are displayed on separate screens, it is awkward and time consuming to click through all of the questions up front to find the FSQs. Therefore, go through the section on a first pass and decide whether to do the passage now or to save it for later, basing your decision on the passage text and the first question. Tackle the FSQs as you come upon them. More details are below.

Here is an outline of the procedure:

1) For each passage, write a heading on your noteboard with the passage number, the general topic, and its range of questions (e.g., "Passage 1, thermodynamics, Q 1–5" or "Passage 2, enzymes, Q 6–9"). The passage numbers do not currently appear in the Navigation or Review screens; thus having the question numbers on your noteboard will allow you to move through the section more efficiently.

2) Skim the text and rank the passage. If a passage is a "Now," complete it before moving on to the next passage (also see Attacking the Questions below). If it is a "Later" passage, first write "SKIPPED" in block letters under the passage heading on your noteboard and leave room for your work when you come back to complete that passage. (Note that the specific passages you skip will be unique to you; in the Bio/Biochem section, you might choose to do all Biology passages first and then come back for Biochemistry. Or in Chem/Phys you might choose to skip experiment-based or analytical passage. Know ahead of time what type of passage you are going to skip and follow your plan.)

3) Next, click on the "Navigation" button at the bottom to get to the Navigation screen. Click on the first question of the next passage; you'll be able to identify it because you know the range of questions from the passage you just skipped. This will take you to the next passage, where you will repeat steps 1–3.

4) Once you have completed the "Now" passages, go to the Review screen and click the first question for the first passage you skipped. Answer the questions, and continue going back to the Review screen and repeating this procedure for other passages you have skipped.

Attacking the Questions

As you work through the questions, if you encounter a particularly lengthy question, or a question that requires a lot of analysis, you may choose to skip it. This is a wise strategy because it ensures you will tackle all the easier questions first, the ones you are more likely to get right. If you choose to skip the question (or if you attempt it but get stuck), write down the question number on your noteboard, click the Flag for Review button to flag the question in the Review screen, and move on to the next question. At the end of the passage, click back through the set of questions to complete any that you skipped over the first time through, and make sure that you have filled in an answer for every question.

General Strategy for the CARS Section

Ranking and Ordering the Passages: What to Start With

Ranking: Since the questions are displayed on separate screens, it is awkward and time consuming to click through all of the questions before ranking each passage as "Now" (an easier passage), "Later" (a harder passage), or "Killer" (a passage that you will randomly guess on). Therefore, rank the passage and decide whether or not to do it on the first pass through the section based on the passage text, skimming the first 2–3 sentences.

Ordering: Because of the additional clicking through screens (or, use of the Review screen) that is required to navigate through the section, the "Two-Pass" system (completing the "Now" passages as you find them) is likely to be your most efficient approach. However, if you find that you are continuously making a lot of bad ranking decisions, it is still valid to experiment with the "Three-Pass" approach (ranking all nine passages up front before attempting your first "Now" passage).

Here is an outline of the basic Ranking and Ordering procedure to follow.

1) For each passage, write a heading on your noteboard with the passage number and its range of questions (e.g. "Passage 1, Q 1–7"). The passage numbers do not currently appear in the Navigation or Review screens, thus having the question numbers on your noteboard will allow you to move through the section more efficiently.

2) Skim the first 2–3 sentences and rank the passage. If the passage is a "Now," complete it before moving on to the next. If it is a "Later" or "Killer," first write either "Later" or "Killer" and "SKIPPED" in block letters under the passage heading on your noteboard and leave room for your work if you decide to come back and complete that passage. Then click through each question, flagging each one and filling in random guesses, until you get to the next passage.

3) Once you have completed the "Now" passages, come back for your second pass and complete the "Later" passages, leaving your random guesses in place for any "Killer" passages that you choose not to complete. Go to the Review screen and use your noteboard notes on the question numbers. Click on the number of the first question for that passage to go back to that question, and proceed from there. Alternatively, if you have consistently flagged all the questions for passages you skipped in your first pass you can use "Review Flagged" from the Review screen to find and complete your "Later" passages.

4) Regardless of how you choose to find your second pass passages, unflag each question after you complete it, so that you can continue to rely on the Review screen (and the "Review Flagged" function) to identify questions that you have not yet attempted.

Previewing the Questions

The formatting and functioning of the tools facilitates effective previewing. Having each question on a separate screen will encourage you to really focus on that question. Even more importantly, you can highlight in the question stem and in the answer choices.

Here is the basic procedure for previewing the questions:

1) Start with the first question, and if it has lead words referencing passage content, highlight them. You may also choose to jot them down on your noteboard. Once you reach and preview the last question for the set on that passage, THEN stay on that screen and work the passage (your highlighting appears and stays on every passage screen, and persists through the whole 90 minutes).

2) Once you have worked the passage and defined the Bottom Line—the main idea and tone of the entire passage—work **backward** from the last question to the first. If you skip over any questions as you go (see Attacking the Questions below), write down the question number on your noteboard. Then click **forward** through the set of questions, completing any that you skipped over the first time through. Once you reach and complete the last question for that passage, clicking "Next" will send you to the first question of the next passage. Working the questions from last to first the first time through the set will eliminate the need to click back through multiple screens to get to the first question immediately after previewing, and it will also make it easier and more efficient to do the hardest questions last (see Attacking the Questions below).

3) Remember that previewing questions is a CARS-only technique. It is not efficient to preview questions in the science sections.

Attacking the Questions

The question types and the procedure for actually attacking each type will be discussed later. However, it is still important **not** to attempt the hardest questions first (potentially getting stuck, wasting time, and discouraging yourself).

So, as you work the questions from last to first (see Previewing the Questions above), if you encounter a particularly difficult and/or lengthy question (or if you attempt a question but get stuck), write down the question number on your noteboard (you may also choose to Flag it) and move on to the next question. Then click **forward** through the set and complete any that you skipped over the first time through the set, unflagging any questions that you flagged that first time through and making sure that you have filled in an answer for every question.

Pacing Strategy for the MCAT

Since the MCAT is a timed test, you must keep an eye on the timer and adjust your pacing as necessary. It would be terrible to run out of time at the end only to discover that the last few questions could have been easily answered in just a few seconds each.

In the science sections, you will have about one minute and thirty-five seconds (1:35) per question, and in the CARS section you will have about one minute and forty seconds (1:40) per question (not taking into account time reading the passage before answering the questions).

Section	# of Questions in Passage	Approximate Time (including reading the passage)
Chem/Phys, Bio/Biochem, and Psych/Soc	4	6.5 minutes
	5	8 minutes
	6	9.5 minutes
CARS	5	8.5 minutes
	6	10 minutes
	7	11.5 minutes

When starting a passage in the science sections, make note of how much time you will allot for it and the starting time on the timer. Jot down on your noteboard what the timer should say at the end of the passage. Then just keep an eye on it as you work through the questions. If you are near the end of the time for that passage, guess on any remaining questions, make some notes on your noteboard, Flag the questions, and move on. Come back to those questions if you have time.

For the CARS section, keep in mind that many people will maximize their score by *not* trying to complete every question or every passage in the section. A good strategy for test takers who cannot achieve a high level of accuracy on all nine passages is to randomly guess on at least one passage in the section, and spend your time getting a high percentage of the other questions right. To complete all nine CARS passages, you have about 10 minutes per passage. To complete eight of the nine, you have about 11 minutes per passage.

To help maximize your number of correct answer choices in any section, do the questions and passages within that section in the order *you* want to do them (see General Strategy).

Process of Elimination

Process of Elimination (POE) is probably the most useful technique you have to tackle MCAT questions. Since there is no guessing penalty, POE allows you to increase your probability of choosing the correct answer by eliminating those you are sure are wrong.

1) Strike out any choices that you are sure are incorrect or that do not address the issue raised in the question.
2) Jot down some notes to help clarify your thoughts if you return to the question.
3) Use the "Flag for Review" button to flag the question for review. (Note, however, that in the CARS section, you generally should not be returning to rethink questions once you have moved on to a new passage.)
4) Do not leave it blank! For the sciences, if you are not sure and you have already spent more than 60 seconds on that question, just pick one of the remaining choices. If you have time to review it at the end, you can always debate the remaining choices based on your previous notes. For CARS, if you have been through the choices two or three times, have reread the question stem and gone back to the passage and you are still stuck, move on. Do the remaining questions for that passage, take one more look at the question you were stuck on, then pick an answer and move on for good.

5) Special Note: If three of the four answer choices have been eliminated, the remaining choice must be the correct answer. Don't waste time pondering *why* it is correct, just click it and move on. The MCAT doesn't care if you truly understand why it's the right answer, only that you have the right answer selected.

6) More subject-specific information on techniques will be presented in the next chapter.

Guessing

Remember, there is NO guessing penalty on the MCAT. NEVER leave a question blank!

QUESTION TYPES

In the science sections of the MCAT, the questions fall into one of three main categories.

1) Memory questions: These questions can be answered directly from prior knowledge and represent about 25 percent of the total number of questions.

2) Explicit questions: These questions are those for which the answer is explicitly stated in the passage. To answer them correctly, for example, may just require finding a definition, reading a graph, or making a simple connection. Explicit questions represent about 35 percent of the total number of questions.

3) Implicit questions: These questions require you to apply knowledge to a new situation; the answer is typically implied by the information in the passage. These questions often start "if…then…." (For example, "If we modify the experiment in the passage like this, then what result would we expect?") Implicit style questions make up about 40 percent of the total number of questions.

In the CARS section, the questions fall into four main categories:

1) Specific questions: These either ask you for facts from the passage (Retrieval questions) or require you to deduce what is most likely to be true based on the passage (Inference questions).

2) General questions: These ask you to summarize themes (Main Idea and Primary Purpose questions) or evaluate an author's opinion (Tone/Attitude questions).

3) Reasoning questions: These ask you to describe the purpose of, or the support provided for, a statement made in the passage (Structure questions) or to judge how well the author supports his or her argument (Evaluate questions).

4) Application questions: These ask you to apply new information to the passage—information from either the question stem itself (New Information questions) or from the answer choices (Strengthen, Weaken, and Analogy questions).

More detail on question types and strategies can be found in Chapter 2.

TESTING TIPS

Before Test Day

- Take a trip to the test center at least a day or two before your actual test date so that you can easily find the building and room on test day. This will also allow you to gauge traffic and see if you need money for parking or anything like that. Knowing this type of information ahead of time will greatly reduce your stress on the day of your test.
- During the week before the test, adjust your sleeping schedule so that you are going to bed and getting up in the morning at the same times as on the day before and morning of the MCAT. Prioritize getting a reasonable amount of sleep during the last few nights before the test.
- Don't do any heavy studying the day before the test. This is not a test you can cram for! Your goal at this point is to rest and relax so that you can go into test day in a good physical and mental condition.
- Eat well. Try to avoid excessive caffeine and sugar. Ideally, in the weeks leading up to the actual test you should experiment a little bit with foods and practice tests to see which foods give you the most endurance. Aim for steady blood sugar levels during the test: sports drinks, peanut-butter crackers, trail mix, etc. make good snacks for your breaks and lunch.

General Test Day Info and Tips

- On the day of the test, arrive at the test center at least a half hour prior to the start time of your test.
- Examinees will be checked in to the center in the order in which they arrive.
- You will be assigned a locker or secure area in which to put your personal items. Textbooks and study notes are not allowed, so there is no need to take them with you to the test center.
- Your ID will be checked, a scan of your palm will be taken, and you will be asked to sign in.
- You will be given a noteboard booklet and a wet-erase marker. The test center administrator will take you to the computer on which you will complete the test. You may not choose a computer; you must use the computer assigned to you.
- Nothing, not even your watch, is allowed at the computer station except your photo ID, your locker key (if provided), and a factory sealed packet of ear plugs.
- If you choose to leave the testing room at the breaks, you will have your palm scanned again, and you will have to sign in and out.
- You are allowed to access the items in your locker, except for notes and cell phones. (Check your test center's policy on cell phones ahead of time; some centers do not even allow them to be kept in your locker.)
- Don't forget to take the snack foods and lunch you experimented with during your practice tests.
- At the end of the test, the test administrator will collect your noteboard and clean off your notes.
- Definitely take the breaks! Get up and walk around. It's a good way to clear your head between sections and get the blood (and oxygen!) flowing to your brain.
- Ask for a clean noteboard at the breaks if you want a fresh one.

Chapter 2
Biochemistry
Strategy for the MCAT

2.1 SCIENCE SECTIONS OVERVIEW

There are three science sections on the MCAT:

- Chemical and Physical Foundations of Biological Systems
- Biological and Biochemical Foundations of Living Systems
- Psychological, Social, and Biological Foundations of Behavior

The Chemical and Physical Foundations of Biological Systems section (Chem/Phys) is the first section on the test. It includes questions from General Chemistry (about 30%), Physics (about 25%), Organic Chemistry (about 15%), Biochemistry (about 25%), and Biology (about 5%). Further, the questions often test chemical and physical concepts within a biological setting: for example, pressure and fluid flow in blood vessels. A solid grasp of math fundamentals is required (arithmetic, algebra, graphs, trigonometry, vectors, proportions, and logarithms); however, there are no calculus-based questions.

The Biological and Biochemical Foundations of Living Systems section (Bio/Biochem) is the third section on the test. Approximately 65% of the questions in this section come from Biology, approximately 25% come from Biochemistry, and approximately 10% come from Organic and General Chemistry. Math calculations are generally not required on this section of the test; however, a basic understanding of statistics as used in biological research is helpful.

The Psychological, Social, and Biological Foundations of Behavior section (Psych/Soc) is the fourth and final section on the test. About 65% of the questions will be drawn from Psychology (and about 5% of these will be Biological Psychology), about 30% from Sociology, and about 5% from Biology. As with the Bio/Biochem section, calculations are generally not required; however a basic understanding of statistics as used in research is helpful.

Most of the questions in the science sections (44 of the 59) are passage-based, and each section has 10 passages. Passages consist of a few paragraphs of information and include equations, reactions, graphs, figures, tables, experiments, and data. Four to six questions will be associated with each passage.

The remaining 25% of the questions (15 of 59) in each science section are freestanding questions (FSQs). These questions appear in approximately four groups interspersed between the passages. Each group contains three to four questions.

You are allowed 95 minutes to complete each of the science sections. This breaks down to approximately one minute and 35 seconds per question.

2.2 SCIENCE PASSAGE TYPES

The passages in the science sections fall into one of three main categories: Information and/or Situation Presentation, Experiment/Research Presentation, or Persuasive Reasoning.

Information and/or Situation Presentation

These passages either present straightforward scientific information or they describe a particular event or occurrence. Generally, questions associated with these passages test basic science facts or ask you to predict outcomes given new variables or new information. Here is an example of an Information/Situation Presentation passage:

Figure 1 shows a portion of the inner mechanism of a typical home smoke detector. It consists of a pair of capacitor plates which are charged by a 9-volt battery (not shown). The capacitor plates (electrodes) are connected to a sensor device, D; the resistor R denotes the internal resistance of the sensor. Normally, air acts as an insulator and no current would flow in the circuit shown. However, inside the smoke detector is a small sample of an artificially produced radioactive element, americium-241, which decays primarily by emitting alpha particles, with a half-life of approximately 430 years. The daughter nucleus of the decay has a half-life in excess of two million years and therefore poses virtually no biohazard.

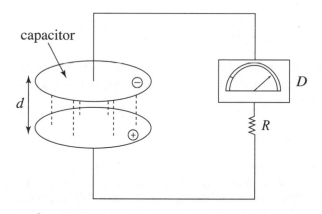

Figure 1 Smoke detector mechanism

The decay products (alpha particles and gamma rays) from the ^{241}Am sample ionize air molecules between the plates and thus provide a conducting pathway which allows current to flow in the circuit shown in Figure 1. A steady-state current is quickly established and remains as long as the battery continues to maintain a 9-volt potential difference between its terminals. However, if smoke particles enter the space between the capacitor plates and thereby interrupt the flow, the current is reduced, and the sensor responds to this change by triggering the alarm. (Furthermore, as the battery starts to "die out," the resulting drop in current is also detected to alert the homeowner to replace the battery.)

$$C = \varepsilon_0 \frac{A}{d}$$

Equation 1

where ε_0 is the universal permittivity constant, equal to 8.85 $\times 10^{-12}$ $C^2/(N\ m^2)$. Since the area A of each capacitor plate in the smoke detector is 20 cm^2 and the plates are separated by a distance d of 5 mm, the capacitance is 3.5×10^{-12} F = 3.5 pF.

Experiment/Research Presentation

These passages present the details of experiments and research procedures. They often include data tables and graphs. Generally, questions associated with these passages ask you to interpret data, draw conclusions, and make inferences. Here is an example of an Experiment/Research Presentation passage:

The development of sexual characteristics depends upon various factors, the most important of which are hormonal control, environmental stimuli, and the genetic makeup of the individual. The hormones that contribute to the development include the steroid hormones estrogen, progesterone, and testosterone, as well as the pituitary hormones FSH (follicle-stimulating hormone) and LH (luteinizing hormone).

To study the mechanism by which estrogen exerts its effects, a researcher performed the following experiments using cell culture assays.

Experiment 1:

Human embryonic placental mesenchyme (HEPM) cells were grown for 48 hours in Dulbecco's Modified Eagle Medium (DMEM), with media change every 12 hours. Upon confluent growth, cells were exposed to a 10 mg per mL solution of green fluorescent-labeled estrogen for 1 hour. Cells were rinsed with DMEM and observed under confocal fluorescent microscopy.

Experiment 2:

HEPM cells were grown to confluence as in Experiment 1. Cells were exposed to Pesticide A for 1 hour, followed by the 10 mg/mL solution of labeled estrogen, rinsed as in Experiment 1, and observed under confocal fluorescent microscopy.

Experiment 3:

Experiment 1 was repeated with Chinese Hamster Ovary (CHO) cells instead of HEPM cells.

Experiment 4:

CHO cells injected with cytoplasmic extracts of HEPM cells were grown to confluence, exposed to the 10 mg/mL solution of labeled estrogen for 1 hour, and observed under confocal fluorescent microscopy.

The results of these experiments are given in Table 1.

Table 1 Detection of Estrogen (+ indicates presence of Estrogen)

Experiment	Media	Cytoplasm	Nucleus
1	+	+	+
2	+	+	+
3	+	+	I
4	+	+	+

After observing the cells in each experiment, the researcher bathed the cells in a solution containing 10 mg per mL of a red fluorescent probe that binds specifically to the estrogen receptor only when its active site is occupied. After 1 hour, the cells were rinsed with DMEM and observed under confocal fluorescent microscopy. The results are presented in Table 2.

The researcher also repeated Experiment 2 using Pesticide B, an estrogen analog, instead of Pesticide A. Results from other researchers had shown that Pesticide B binds to the active site of the cytosolic estrogen receptor (with an affinity 10,000 times greater than that of estrogen) and causes increased transcription of mRNA.

Table 2 Observed Fluorescence and Estrogen Effects (G = green, R = red)

Experiment	Media	Cytoplasm	Nucleus	Estrogen effects observed?
1	G only	G and R	G and R	Yes
2	G only	G only	G only	No
3	G only	G only	G only	No
4	G only	G and R	G and R	Yes

Based on these results, the researcher determined that estrogen had no effect when not bound to a cytosolic, estrogen-specific receptor.

Persuasive Reasoning

These passages typically present a scientific phenomenon along with a hypothesis that explains the phenomenon, and may include counter-arguments as well. Questions associated with these passages ask you to evaluate the hypothesis or arguments. Persuasive Reasoning passages in the science sections of the MCAT tend to be less common than Information Presentation or Experiment/Research Presentation passages. Here is an example of a Persuasive Reasoning passage:

Two theoretical chemists attempted to explain the observed trends of acidity by applying two interpretations of molecular orbital theory. Consider the pK_a values of some common acids listed along with the conjugate base:

acid	pK_a	conjugate base
H_2SO_4	< 0	HSO_4^-
H_2CrO_4	5.0	$HCrO_4^-$
H_2PO_4	2.1	$H_2PO_4^-$
HF	3.9	F^-
HOCl	7.8	ClO^-
HCN	9.5	CN^-
HIO_3	1.2	IO_3^-

Recall that acids with a $pK_a < 0$ are called strong acids, and those with a $pK_a > 0$ are called weak acids. The arguments of the chemists are given below.

Chemist #1:

"The acidity of a compound is proportional to the polarization of the H—X bond, where X is some nonmetal element. Complex acids, such as H_2SO_4, $HClO_4$, and HNO_3 are strong acids because the H—O bonding electrons are strongly drawn towards the oxygen. It is generally true that a covalent bond weakens as its polarization increases. Therefore, one can conclude that the strength of an acid is proportional to the number of electronegative atoms in that acid."

Chemist #2:

"The acidity of a compound is proportional to the number of stable resonance structures of that acid's conjugate base. H_2SO_4, $HClO_4$, and HNO_3 are all strong acids because their respective conjugate bases exhibit a high degree of resonance stabilization."

Mapping a Passage

"Mapping a passage" refers to the combination of on-screen highlighting and noteboard notes that you take while working through a passage. Typically, good things to highlight include the overall topic of a paragraph, unfamiliar terms, italicized terms, unusual terms, numerical values, any hypothesis, and experimental results. Noteboard notes can be used to summarize the paragraphs and to jot down important facts and connections that are made when reading the passage. More details on passage mapping will be presented in Section 2.5.

2.3 SCIENCE QUESTION TYPES

Questions in the science sections are generally one of three main types: Memory, Explicit, or Implicit.

Memory Questions

These questions can be answered directly from prior knowledge, with no need to reference the passage or question text. Memory questions represent approximately 25 percent of the science questions on the MCAT. Usually, Memory questions are found as FSQs, but they can also be tucked into a passage. Here's an example of a Memory question:

Which of the following acetylating conditions will convert diethylamine into an amide at the fastest rate?

A) Acetic acid / HCl
B) Acetic anhydride
C) Acetyl chloride
D) Ethyl acetate

Explicit Questions

Explicit questions can be answered primarily with information from the passage, along with prior knowledge. They may require data retrieval, graph analysis, or making a simple connection. Explicit questions make up approximately 35–40 percent of the science questions on the MCAT; here's an example (taken from the Information/Situation Presentation passage):

The sensor device D shown in Figure 1 performs its function by acting as:

A) an ohmmeter.
B) a voltmeter.
C) a potentiometer.
D) an ammeter.

Implicit Questions

These questions require you to take information from the passage, combine it with your prior knowledge, apply it to a new situation, and come to some logical conclusion. They typically require more complex connections than do Explicit questions, and they may also require data retrieval, graph analysis, etc. Implicit questions usually require a solid understanding of the passage information. They make up approximately 35–40 percent of the science questions on the MCAT; here's an example (taken from the Experiment/Research Presentation passage):

If Experiment 2 were repeated, but this time exposing the cells first to Pesticide A and then to Pesticide B before exposing them to the green fluorescent-labeled estrogen and the red fluorescent probe, which of the following statements will most likely be true?

A) Pesticide A and Pesticide B bind to the same site on the estrogen receptor.
B) Estrogen effects would be observed.
C) Only green fluorescence would be observed.
D) Both green and red fluorescence would be observed.

The Rod of Asclepius

You may notice this Rod of Asclepius icon as you read through the book. In Greek mythology, the Rod of Asclepius is associated with healing and medicine; the symbol continues to be used today to represent medicine and healthcare. You won't see this on the actual MCAT, but we've used it here to call attention to medically related examples and questions.

2.4 BIOCHEMISTRY ON THE MCAT

The science sections of the MCAT all have 59 questions: 10 passages (with 44 total questions) and 15 freestanding questions. Biochemistry makes up a sizable chunk of two different sections of the MCAT. 25% of the Chemical and Physical Foundations of Biological Systems section, and 25% of the Biological and Biochemical Foundations of Living Systems section are made up of Biochemistry passages and questions. This means that in both sections approximately 15 of the 59 questions will be biochemistry based, and likely 2–3 of the passages will have a biochemistry theme. The application of this material can be anything from the details of some biochemical pathway, to the complexities of an experiment on a novel drug, to the subtleties of a condition caused by a missing or malfunctioning enzyme.

2.5 TACKLING A BIOCHEMISTRY PASSAGE

Generally speaking, time is not an issue in the Bio/Biochem section of the MCAT. Because students have a stronger background in biology and biochemistry than in other subjects, the passages seem more understandable; in fact, readers sometimes find themselves getting caught up and interested in the passage. Often, students report having about 5 to 10 minutes "left over" after completing the section. This means that an additional minute or so can potentially be spent on each passage, thinking and understanding.

Passage Types as They Apply to Biochemistry

Experiment/Research Presentation: Biochemistry

This is the most common type of Biochemistry passage. It typically presents the details behind an experiment along with data tables, graphs, and figures. Often these are the most difficult passages to deal with because they require an understanding of the reasoning behind the experiment, the logic to each step, and the ability to analyze the results and form conclusions. A basic understanding of biometry (basic statistics as they apply to biology and biochemistry research) is necessary.

Information/Situation Presentation: Biochemistry

This is the second most common type of Biochemistry passage on the MCAT. These passages generally appear as one of two variants: either a basic concept with additional levels of detail included (for example, all the detail you ever wanted to know about the electron transport chain), or a novel concept with ties to basic information (for example, a rare inborn error of metabolism and its effect on the body). Either way, Biochemistry passages are notorious for testing concepts in unusual contexts. The key to dealing with these passages is to, first, not become anxious about all the stuff you might not know, and second, figure out how the basics you do know apply to the new situation. For example, you might be presented with a passage that introduces hormones you never heard of or novel drugs to combat diseases you didn't know existed. First, don't panic. Second, look for how these new things fit into familiar categories: for example, "peptide vs. steroid" or "competitive inhibitor." Then answer the questions with these basics in mind.

That said, you have to know your basics. This will increase your confidence in answering freestanding questions, as well as increase the speed with which to find the information in the passage. The astute MCAT student will never waste time staring at a question thinking, "Should I know this?" Instead, because she has a solid understanding of the necessary core knowledge, she'll say, "No, I am NOT expected to know this, and I am going to look for it in the passage."

2.5

Persuasive Reasoning: Biochemistry

This is the least common passage type in Biochemistry. It typically describes some biological or biochemical phenomenon and offers one or more theories to explain it. Questions in Persuasive Reasoning passages ask you to determine support for one of the theories or present new evidence and ask which theory is now contradicted.

One last thought about Biochemistry passages in general: because the array of topics is so vast, passages in these sections of the test often pull questions from multiple areas of biology and/or biochemistry into a single, general topic. Consider, for example, a passage on hemoglobin. Question topics could include basics about enzymes and cooperative binding, protein structure, DNA mutations, effects of sickle cell disease, regulation of expression of the hemoglobin genes, and the data from an experiment done on sickle cell patients.

Reading a Biochemistry Passage

Although tempting, try not to get bogged down reading all the little details in a passage. Again, because most premeds have an inherent interest in biology and the mechanisms behind disease, it's very easy to get lost in the science behind the passages. In spite of having that "extra" time, you don't want to use it all up reading what isn't necessary. Each passage type requires a slightly different style of reading.

Information/Situation Presentation passages require the least reading. These should be skimmed to get an idea of the location of information within the passage. These passages include a fair amount of detail that you might not need, so save the reading of these details until a question comes up about them. Then go back and read for the finer nuances.

Experiment/Research Presentation passages require the most reading. You are practically guaranteed to get questions that ask you about the details of the experiment, why a particular step was carried out, why the results are what they are, how to interpret the data, or how the results might change if a particular variable is altered. It's worth spending a little more time reading to understand the experiment. However, because there will be a fair number of questions unrelated to the experiment, you might consider answering these first and then going back for the experiment details.

Persuasive Argument passages are somewhere in the middle. You can skim them for location of information, but you also want to spend a little time reading the details of and thinking about the arguments presented. It is extremely likely that you will be asked a question about them.

Advanced Reading Skills

To improve your ability to read and glean information from a passage, you need to practice. Be critical when you read the content; watch for vague areas or holes in the passage that aren't explained clearly. Remember that information about new topics will be woven throughout the passage; you may need to piece together information from several paragraphs and a figure to get the whole picture.

After you've read, highlighted, and mapped a passage (more on this in a bit), stop and ask yourself the following questions:

- What was this passage about? What was the conclusion or main point?
- Was there a paragraph that was mostly background?
- Were there paragraphs or figures that seemed useless?
- What information was found in each paragraph? Why was that paragraph there?
- Are there any holes in the story?
- What extra information could I have pulled out of the passage? What inferences or conclusions could I make?
- If something unique was explained or mentioned, what might be its purpose?
- What am I *not* being told?
- Can I summarize the purpose and/or results of the experiment in a few sentences?
- Were there any comparisons in the passage?

This takes awhile at first, but eventually it will become second nature and you'll start doing it as you read the passage. If you have a study group you are working with, consider doing this as an exercise with your study partners. Take turns asking and answering the questions above. Having to explain something to someone else not only solidifies your own knowledge, but helps you see where you might be weak.

Mapping a Biochemistry Passage

Mapping a Biochemistry passage is a combination of highlighting and noteboard notes that can help you organize and understand the passage information.

Resist the temptation to highlight everything! (Everyone has done this: you're reading a textbook with a highlighter, and then look back and realize that the whole page is yellow!) Restrict your highlighting to a few things:

- the main theme of a paragraph
- an unusual or unfamiliar term that is defined specifically for that passage (e.g., something that is italicized)
- statements that either support the main theme or contradict the main theme
- list topics: sometimes lists appear in paragraph form within a passage. Highlight the general topic of the list.
- relationships (how one thing changes relative to another thing)

The noteboard should be organized. Make sure the passage number appears at the top of your noteboard notes. For each paragraph, note "P1," "P2," etc., on the noteboard, and jot down a few notes about that paragraph. Try to translate biology/biochemistry jargon into your own words using everyday language (this is particularly useful for experiments). Also, make sure to note down simple relationships (e.g., the relationship between two variables).

Pay attention to equations, figures, and the like to see what type of information they deal with. Don't spend a lot of time analyzing at this point, but do jot down on your noteboard "Fig 1" and a brief summary of the data. Also, if you've discovered a list in the passage, note its topic and location on your noteboard.

Let's take a look at how we might highlight and map a passage. Below is a passage on the pentose phosphate pathway.

The pentose phosphate pathway (PPP) produces ribose-5-phosphate from glucose-6-phosphate and generates NADPH, which is used by the cell in biosynthetic pathways (such as fatty acid biosynthesis) as a reducing agent. Ribose-5-phosphate is converted to 5-phosphoribosyl-1-pyrophosphate (PRPP) by the enzyme ribose phosphate pyrophosphokinase. PRPP is an essential precursor in the biosynthesis of all nucleotides. Ribose phosphate pyrophosphokinase is inhibited by both ADP and GDP nucleotides.

The committed step in purine nucleotide synthesis is catalyzed by the enzyme amidophosphoribosyl transferase, which uses glutamine and PRPP as substrates. This enzyme is inhibited by AMP and GMP and is activated by high concentrations of PRPP. An intermediate in purine biosynthesis is inosine monophosphate (IMP). The conversion of IMP to AMP is inhibited by AMP, and the conversion of IMP to GMP is inhibited by GMP. An essential precursor in pyrimidine biosynthesis is carbamoyl phosphate, which is generated by the enzyme carbamoyl phosphate synthase. This enzyme is inhibited by UTP and activated by ATP and PRPP. The production of CTP from UTP is inhibited by CTP. These reactions are summarized in Figure 1.

2.5

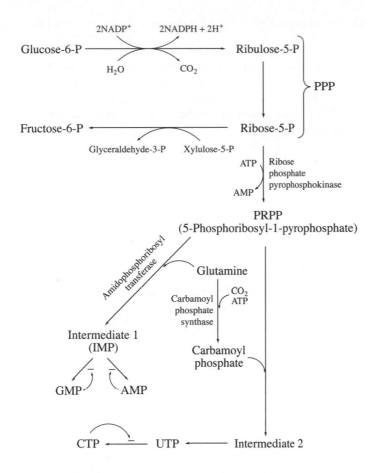

Figure 1 Biosynthetic pathway

Analysis and Passage Map

This passage is an Information Presentation passage and starts out with a paragraph about the pentose phosphate pathway. This is primarily a background paragraph and can be skimmed quickly, with a few words highlighted.

The second paragraph goes into more detail about the steps in purine and pyrimidine biosynthesis and specifically discusses some of the enzymes and their inhibitors. This paragraph presents information that is beyond what you are expected to know about the pentose phosphate pathway for the MCAT. Figure 1 shows some of the details of the pathway.

Here's what your passage map might look like:

> P1 – *pentose phosphate pathway, products and their uses*
> P2 – *committed step purines, enzyme and inhib.*
> *precursor to pyrim., enzyme, and inhib.*
> *Fig 1 = details of pathway*

Let's take a look at a different passage. Below is an Experiment/Research Presentation passage.

In times of fasting, the body relies more heavily on catabolism of amino acids to produce either ketone bodies (in the case of ketogenic amino acids) or precursors of glucose (in the case of glucogenic amino acids) through a series of interactions involving an α-ketoacid intermediate. A representative reaction is shown in Figure 1.

glutamate   pyruvate

α-ketoglutarate   alanine

Figure 1   Interconversion of pyruvate and alanine

"Low carb" diets capitalize on this feature of metabolism to achieve a ketogenic state in which the body is chronically deprived of carbohydrate sources of energy and thus forced to produce ketone bodies from either fat or amino acids to obtain energy. Interested in changes in the makeup of energy molecules in blood during this ketogenic state, researchers measure the levels of ketone bodies, glucose, insulin, glucagon, and fatty acids at various time points after a participant begins a ketogenic diet. Their findings are shown below.

	After normal meal	Overnight fasting	2 days after starting diet	5 days after starting diet
Insulin	↑	↓	↓	↓
Glucagon	↓	↑	↑	↑
Glucose	Normal	Normal	Normal	Normal
Fatty Acids	↑	↓	↑	↑↑↑
Ketones	↓	↓	↑	↑↑↑

Figure 2   Results of experiment

Adapted from Harvey, R. A., & Ferrier, D. R. (2011). *Lippincott's illustrated reviews, biochemistry* (5th ed.). Philadelphia: Wolters Kluwer Health.

Analysis and Passage Map

This passage starts out by describing the effects of fasting on the body and how it turns to amino acid catabolism to generate ketones or glucose precursors. It mentions the involvement of an α-ketoacid intermediate; Figure 1 shows this reaction.

The second paragraph describes how "low carb" diets can lead to ketogenesis. It also describes the experiment and refers us to Figure 2 for the results of the experiment.

Here's how your map might look:

> P1 – fasting, a.a. catabolism → ketones, glu precursors
> P2 – low carb diet effects, desc. of experiment
> Fig 2 – keto diet causes ↑ glucagon, fats, and ketones and ↓ insulin

One last thought about passages: as with all sections on the MCAT, you can do the passages in the order *you* want to. There are no extra points for taking the test in order. Generally, passages in the Bio/Biochem section will fall into one of four main subject groups:

- biochemistry
- other non-physiology
- physiology
- organic/general chemistry

Figure out which group you are most comfortable with and do those passages first. See Chapter 1 for general strategies for moving through each of the sections efficiently.

2.5

2.6 TACKLING THE QUESTIONS

Questions in the Bio/Biochem section mimic the three typical questions of the science sections in general: Memory, Explicit, and Implicit.

Question Types as They Apply to Biochemistry

Biochemistry Memory Questions

Memory questions are exactly what they sound like: they test your knowledge of some specific fact or concept. While Memory questions are typically found as freestanding questions, they can also be tucked into a passage. These questions, aside from requiring memorization, do not generally cause problems for students because they are similar to the types of questions that appear on a typical college biochemistry exam. Below is an example of a freestanding Memory question:

> ACE inhibitors are a class of drugs frequently prescribed to treat hypertension. Captopril, a compound that is structurally similar to angiotensin I, was developed in 1975 as the first ACE inhibitor. When patients take Captopril, which of the following is true about the kinetics of their ACE?
>
> A) V_{max} decreases, K_m remains the same.
> B) V_{max} remains the same, K_m increases.
> C) Both V_{max} and K_m increase.
> D) Both V_{max} and K_m remain the same.

The correct answer to the question above is choice B. Here's another example. This question is from a passage:

> GAPDH converts an aldehyde into a carboxylic acid in order to change NAD^+ to NADH. Which of the following is true regarding this reaction in humans?
>
> A) The aldehyde is reduced.
> B) NAD^+ is oxidized.
> C) NAD^+ gains 2 e^- and one proton.
> D) The carboxylic acid ($pK_a = 2.19$) is mostly in its protonated form.

The question asks you to draw on your knowledge of oxidation/reduction reactions. The correct answer is choice C.

There is no specific "trick" to answering Memory questions; either you know the answer or you don't.

If you find that you are missing a fair number of Memory questions, it is a sure sign that you don't know the content well enough. Go back and review.

Biochemistry Explicit Questions

True, pure Explicit questions are rare in the Bio/Biochem section. A purely Explicit question can be answered only with information in the passage. Below is an example of a pure Explicit question taken from the previous pentose phosphate pathway passage:

Which of the following are products of the pentose phosphate pathway?

   I.   NADPH
   II. Glycolytic intermediates
  III. Ribose-5-phosphate

A) I only
B) II only
C) I and III only
D) I, II, and III

The map for this passage indicates that information about the products of the pathway are in paragraph 1 and Figure 1. Paragraph 1 states that NADPH and ribose 5-phosphate are both products, and Figure 1 shows that both fructose 6-P and glyceraldehyde 3-P are glycolytic intermediates. The correct answer is choice D.

However, more often in this section, Explicit questions are more of a blend of Explicit and Memory; they require not only retrieval of passage information, but also recall of some relevant fact. They usually do not require a lot of analysis or connections. Here's an example of the more common type of Explicit question, taken from the ketogenesis passage on page 28:

Which of the following enzymes in the liver is most active five days after someone starts a ketogenic diet?

A) Hexokinase
B) Phosphofructokinase I
C) HMG-CoA synthase
D) Glycogen phosphorylase

To answer this question, you first need to retrieve information from the passage about the substances that are elevated in the blood after five days on a ketogenic diet. From Figure 2 you know that fatty acids, ketones, and glucagon are elevated. You also need to remember the metabolic pathways in which the enzymes in the answer choices participate. Hexokinase and phosphofructokinase I are glycolytic enzymes, and fats and ketones are not products of glycolysis. Thus it is unlikely that these enzymes would be very active (choices A and B can be eliminated). Glycogen phosphorylase breaks down glycogen. Fats and ketones are not the products of glycogen breakdown, so it is unlikely that glycogen phosphorylase would be very active. The correct answer is HMG-CoA synthase, choice C.

Graph interpretation questions comprise a final subgroup in the Explicit question category. These fall into one of two types: those that ask you to take graphical information from the passage and convert it to a text answer, or those that take text from the passage and ask you to convert it to a graph. On the following page is an example of the latter type.

2.6

Which of the following represents the Lineweaver-Burk plot of an enzyme alone (solid line) and in the presence of an inhibitor that binds exclusively to the enzyme active site (dashed line)?

A)

B)

C)

D)

The passage for this question describes how a Lineweaver-Burk plot is generated. You have to combine that information with your knowledge about enzyme inhibitors and how they affect V_{max} and K_m. The correct answer for this question is choice B.

If you find that you are missing Explicit questions, practice your passage mapping. Make sure you aren't missing the critical items in the passage that lead you to the right answer. Slow down a little; take an extra 15 to 30 seconds per passage to read or think about it more carefully.

Biochemistry Implicit Questions

Implicit questions require the most thought. These require recall not only of biochemistry information but also information gleaned from the passage and a more in-depth analysis of how the two relate. Implicit questions require more analysis and connections to be made than Explicit questions. Often they take the form "If...then...." Below is an example of a classic Implicit question, taken from the ketogenesis passage shown earlier.

> If the researchers observed on Day 6 that the levels of fatty acids and ketones decreased while the level of insulin increased, which of the following could be assumed?
>
> A) Protein and amino acid catabolism has increased in this participant.
> B) The participant consumed a meal containing carbohydrates.
> C) An increase in Krebs cycle activity would also be observed.
> D) Glucagon levels would be unchanged from their levels five days after starting the ketogenic diet.

To answer this question, conclusions have to be drawn from the experiments described in the passage, and new conclusions have to be predicted based on the new circumstance. You must make many more connections than when you are answering an Explicit question. From the passage, you need to realize that the low insulin levels on Day 5, combined with high fatty acid and ketone levels in the blood, indicate that the participant is in ketosis, i.e, is burning fat as fuel. If insulin levels suddenly rise while fats and ketones fall, the participant must have eaten some carbohydrates. Protein and amino acid catabolism can result in ketone body production, according to the passage. If protein and amino acid catabolism had increased, you would expect if anything, to see an increase in ketone bodies, not a decrease (choice A is false). There is no reason to assume that Krebs cycle activity would increase; Krebs generally runs well during ketogenesis because of the acetyl CoA from fat breakdown. If the levels of fats are decreased on Day 6, then Krebs cycle activity would likely decrease as well (choice C is false). Insulin and glucagon are opposing hormones; insulin is released when blood sugar levels increase, and glucagon is released when blood sugar levels fall. If insulin is elevated, the glucagon will be decreased (choice D is false).

If you find that you are missing a lot of Implicit questions, first make sure that you are using POE aggressively. Second, go back and review the explanations for the correct answer to figure out where your logic went awry. Did you miss an important fact in the passage? Did you forget the relevant Biochemistry content? Did you follow the logical train of thought to the right answer? Once you figure out where you made your mistake, you will know how to correct it.

2.7 SUMMARY OF THE APPROACH TO BIOCHEMISTRY

How to Map the Passage and Use the Noteboard

1) The passage should not be read like textbook material, with the intent of learning something from every sentence (science majors especially will be tempted to read this way). Passages should be read to get a feel for the type of questions that will follow and to get a general idea of the location of information within the passage.

2) Highlighting—Use this tool sparingly, or you will end up with a passage that is completely covered in yellow highlighter! Highlighting in a Biochemistry passage should be used to draw attention to a few words that demonstrate one of the following:
   - the main theme of a paragraph
   - an unusual or unfamiliar term that is defined specifically for that passage (e.g., something that is italicized)
   - statements that either support the main theme or counteract the main theme
   - list topics (see below)
   - relationships`

3) Pay brief attention to equations, figures, and experiments, noting only what information they deal with. Do not spend a lot of time analyzing at this point.

4) For each passage, start by noting the passage number, the general topic, and the range of questions on your noteboard. You can then work between your noteboard and the Review screen to easily get to the questions you want (see Chapter 1).

5) For each paragraph, note "P1," "P2," etc. on the noteboard and jot down a few notes about that paragraph. Try to translate biochemistry jargon into your own words using everyday language. Especially note down simple relationships (e.g., the relationship between two variables).

6) Lists—Whenever a list appears in paragraph form, jot down on the noteboard the paragraph and the general topic of the list. It will make returning to the passage more efficient and help to organize your thoughts.

7) The noteboard is useful only if it is kept organized! Make sure that your notes for each passage are clearly delineated and marked with the passage number and question range. This will allow you to easily read your notes when you come back to a review a flagged question. Resist the temptation to write in the first available blank space as this makes it much more difficult to refer back to your work.

Biochemistry Question Strategies

1) Remember that the amount of potential content in Biochemistry is significant, so don't panic if something seems completely unfamiliar. Understand the basic content well, find the basics in the unfamiliar topic, and apply them to the question.

2) Process of Elimination is paramount! The strikeout tool allows you to eliminate answer choices; this will improve your chances of guessing the correct answer if you are unable to narrow it down to one choice.

3) Answer the straightforward questions first (typically the memory questions). Leave questions that require analysis of experiments and graphs for later. Take the test in the order YOU want. Make sure to use your noteboard to indicate questions you skipped.

4) Make sure that the answer you choose actually answers the question and isn't just a true statement.

5) Try to avoid answer choices with extreme words such as "always," "never," etc. In biology, there is almost always an exception and answers are rarely black-and-white.

6) Roman numeral questions: whenever possible, start by evaluating the Roman numeral item that shows up in exactly two answer choices. This allows you to quickly eliminate two wrong answer choices regardless of whether the item is true or false. Typically then, you will have to assess only one of the other Roman numeral items to determine the correct answer. Always work between the I-II-III items and the answer choices. Once an item is found to be true (or false), strike out answer choices which do not contain (or do contain) that item number. Make sure to strike out the actual Roman numeral item as well, and highlight those items that are true.

7) LEAST/EXCEPT/NOT questions: don't get tricked by these questions that ask you to pick that answer that doesn't fit (the incorrect or false statement). Make sure to highlight the words "LEAST," "EXCEPT," OR "NOT" in the question stem. It's often good to use your noteboard and write "A B C D" with a T or F next to each answer choice. The one that stands out as different is the correct answer!

8) Again, don't leave any question blank.

A Note About Flashcards

For most of the exams you've taken previously, flashcards were likely very helpful. This was because those exams mostly required you to regurgitate information, and flashcards are pretty good at helping you memorize facts. However, the most challenging aspect of the MCAT is not that it requires you to memorize the fine details of content knowledge, but that it requires you to apply your basic scientific knowledge to unfamiliar situations: flashcards alone may not help you there.

Flashcards can be beneficial if your basic content knowledge is deficient in some area. For example, if you don't know the amino acids and their 1- and 3-letter abbreviations, flashcards can certainly help you memorize these facts. Or, maybe you are unsure of the functions of the different types of enzymes. You might find that flashcards can help you memorize these. But unless you are trying to memorize basic facts in your personal weak areas, you are better off doing and analyzing practice passages than carrying around a stack of flashcards.

Chapter 3
Biochemistry Basics

The notion of life refers to both the activities and the physical structures of living organisms. Both the storage/utilization of energy and the synthesis of structures depend on a large number of chemical reactions that occur within each cell. Fortunately, these reactions do not proceed on their own spontaneously, without regulation. If they did, each cell's energy would rapidly dissipate and total disorder would result. Most reactions are slowed by a large barrier known as the activation energy (E_a), discussed below. The E_a is a bottleneck in a reaction, like a nearly closed gate. The role of the enzyme is to open this chemical gate. In this sense, the enzyme is like a switch. When the enzyme is on, the gate is open (low E_a) and the reaction accelerates. When the enzyme is off, the gate closes and the reaction slows. Before we discuss how enzymes work, we must digress a bit to review the basics of thermodynamics. Then we can review some of the major metabolic pathways in the cell.

3.1 THERMODYNAMICS

Thermodynamics is the study of the energetics of chemical reactions. There are two relevant forms of energy in chemistry: kinetic energy (movement of molecules) and potential energy (energy stored in chemical bonds). [What is the most important potential energy storage molecule in all cells?[1]] The **first law of thermodynamics,** also known as the **law of conservation of energy**, states that the energy of the universe is constant. It implies that when the energy of a system *decreases*, the energy of the rest of the universe (the **surroundings**) must *increase*, and vice versa. The **second law of thermodynamics** states that the disorder, or **entropy,** of the universe tends to increase. Another way to state the second law is as follows: spontaneous reactions tend to increase the disorder of the universe. The symbol for entropy is S, and "a change in entropy" is denoted ΔS, where $\Delta S = S_{final} - S_{initial}$. [If the ΔS of a system is negative, has the disorder of that system increased or decreased?[2]]

A practical way to discuss thermodynamics is the mathematical notion of **free energy** (**Gibbs free energy**), defined by Josiah Gibbs as follows:[3]

$$\textbf{Eq. 1} \quad \Delta G = \Delta H - T\Delta S$$

T denotes temperature, and H denotes **enthalpy**, which is defined by another equation:

$$\textbf{Eq. 2} \quad \Delta H = \Delta E + P\Delta V$$

Here E represents the bond energy of products or reactants in a system, P is pressure, and V is volume. [Given that cellular reactions take place in the liquid phase, how is H related to E in a cell?[4]] ΔG increases with increasing ΔH (bond energy) and decreases with increasing entropy.

- Given the second law of thermodynamics and the mathematical definition of ΔG, which reaction will be favorable: one with a decrease in free energy ($\Delta G < 0$) or one with an increase in free energy ($\Delta G > 0$)?[5]

The change in the Gibbs free energy of a reaction determines whether the reaction is favorable (**spontaneous**, ΔG negative) or unfavorable (**nonspontaneous**, ΔG positive). In terms of the generic reaction

$$A + B \rightarrow C + D$$

the Gibbs free energy change determines whether the reactants (denoted A and B) will stay as they are or be converted to products (C and D).

---

[1] ATP, which stores energy in the ester bonds between its phosphate groups.

[2] If ΔS is negative, then the system lost entropy, which means that disorder decreased.

[3] As in ΔS, the Greek letter Δ (delta) indicates "the change in." For example, $\Delta G_{rxn} = G_{products} - G_{reactants}$.

[4] $H \approx E$, since the change in volume is negligible ($\Delta V \approx 0$).

[5] Favorable reactions have $\Delta G < 0$. We can deduce this from the second law and Equation 1 because the second law states that increasing entropy is favorable, and the equation has ΔG directly related to $-T\Delta S$.

Spontaneous reactions, ones that occur without a net addition of energy, have $\Delta G < 0$. They occur with energy to spare. Reactions with a negative ΔG are **exergonic** (energy *exits* the system); reactions with a positive ΔG are **endergonic**. Endergonic reactions occur only if energy is added. In the lab, energy is added in the form of heat; in the body, endergonic reactions are driven by reaction coupling to exergonic reactions (more on this later). Reactions with a negative ΔH are called **exothermic** and liberate heat. Most metabolic reactions are exothermic (which is how homeothermic organisms such as mammals maintain a constant body temperature). Reactions with a positive ΔH require an input of heat and are referred to as **endothermic**. (Thermodynamics will be discussed in more detail in *MCAT General Chemistry Review* and *MCAT Physics and Math Review*.)

The signs of thermodynamic quantities are assigned from the point of view of *the system*, not the surroundings or the universe. Thus, a negative ΔG means that the system goes to a lower free energy state, and a system will always move in the direction of the lowest free energy. As an analogy, visualize a spinning top as the system. What happens to the top? Does it spin faster and faster? No. It moves towards the lowest energy state. Let's expand the analogy, using an equation:

$$\text{motionless top} \;\rightarrow\; \text{spinning top}$$

Here the "reactant" is the motionless top, and the "product" is the spinning top. Which is lower: the free energy of product or reactant? The reactant. Is the reaction "spontaneous" as written? No; in fact, the reverse reaction is spontaneous. Therefore,

$$G_{\text{spinning}} > G_{\text{motionless}}$$

and thus,

$$\Delta G_{\text{reaction as written (motionless to spinning; left to right)}} > 0$$

So the reaction is nonspontaneous. In other words, *it requires energy input*, namely, energy from your muscles as you spin the top. [If the products in a reaction have more entropy than the reactants and the enthalpy (H) of the reactants and the products are the same, can the reaction occur spontaneously?[6]]

The value of ΔG depends on the concentrations of reactants and products, which can be variable in the body. Therefore, to compare reactions, chemists calculate a standard free energy change, denoted $\Delta G°$, with all reactants and products present at 1 M concentration. Under physiological conditions, however, the hydrogen ion concentration is far from 1 M, so biochemists use an even more standardized ΔG, with 1 M concentration for all solutes except H^+ and a pH of 7; this is denoted $\Delta G°'$.

$\Delta G°'$ is related to the equilibrium constant for a reaction by the following equation:

$$\textbf{Eq. 3} \quad \Delta G°' = -RT \ln K'_{\text{eq}}$$

---

[6] Yes. If $\Delta S > 0$ and $\Delta H = 0$, then according to the second law of thermodynamics, the reaction is spontaneous; see Equation 1.

where R is the gas constant (which would be given on the MCAT, along with the entire equation), and K'_{eq} is the ratio of products to reactants at equilibrium:

$$K'_{eq} = \frac{[C]_{eq}[D]_{eq}}{[A]_{eq}[B]_{eq}}$$

K'_{eq} is the ratio of products to reactants when enough time has passed for equilibrium to be reached [When $K'_{eq} = 1$, what is $\Delta G^{\circ\prime}$?[7]]

But what if we wanted to calculate ΔG for a reaction in the body? In this case, we need one more equation:

Eq. 4 $\Delta G = \Delta G^{\circ\prime} + RT \ln Q$, where $Q = \dfrac{[C][D]}{[A][B]}$

Here, Q is calculated using the actual concentrations of A, B, C, and D (for example, the concentrations in the cell). Equation 4 is simply a conversion from $\Delta G^{\circ\prime}$ (the laboratory standard ΔG with initial concentrations at 1 M) to the real-life here-and-now ΔG. Note that if we put 1 M concentrations of A, B, C, and D into a beaker (at pH 7), we have recreated the laboratory standard initial set-up: $Q = 1$, so $\ln Q = 0$, which means $\Delta G = \Delta G^{\circ\prime}$.

Remember that Q and K_{eq} are not the same. Q is the ratio of products to reactants in any given set-up; K_{eq} is the ratio *at equilibrium*. **Equilibrium** is defined as the point at which the rate of reaction in the forward direction equals the rate of reaction in the reverse direction. At equilibrium, there is constant product and reactant turnover as reactants form products and vice versa, but overall concentrations stay the same. Theoretically (given enough time), all reactant/product systems in a closed system will eventually reach this point.

While all reactions will eventually reach an equilibrium defined by the constant above, we can disturb this balance with the addition or removal of a reactant or product. This causes a change in Q but not K_{eq}, and the reaction will proceed in the direction necessary to reestablish equilibrium. (The shift to restore equilibrium is a demonstration of Le Châtelier's principle which will be discussed in further detail in *MCAT General Chemistry Review*.) Using this principle, a reaction which favors reactants at equilibrium can be driven to generate additional products (such strategies are employed frequently in cellular respiration).

- You are studying a particular reaction. You find the reaction in a book and read $\Delta G^{\circ\prime}$ from a table. Can you calculate ΔG for this reaction in a living human being without any more information?[8]

---

[7] Equation 3 says that $\Delta G^{\circ\prime} = 0$ when $K'_{eq} = 1$ since $\ln 1 = 0$. Note: for more information about MCAT Math, see *MCAT Physics and Math Review*.

[8] No. You need to know the concentrations of A, B, C, and D in the human cell. For example, $\Delta G^{\circ\prime}$ might be +14.8 kcal/mol, indicating that the reaction is very unfavorable under standard conditions and has a $K < 1$, which means that at equilibrium there are more reactants than products. If, however, the ratio of reactants to products is made to be higher than that established at equilibrium, the Q for the reaction becomes less than K, and the forward reaction is spontaneous under these conditions, since ΔG will be less than zero (even though $\Delta G^{\circ\prime}$ will not change). The significance of Q as an independent variable in Equation 4 is that it accounts for Le Châtelier's principle. If a system at equilibrium has reactants added to it, $Q < K$ and $\Delta G < 0$, so the high concentration of reactants will drive the reaction forward to reestablish equilibrium. If a system at equilibrium has products added to it, $Q > K$ and $\Delta G > 0$, so the high concentration of products will drive the reaction backward to reestablish equilibrium. All reactions at equilibrium will respond to these stresses in the same way, regardless of the sign of their $\Delta G^{\circ\prime}$.

- How can ΔG be negative if $\Delta G^{\circ\prime}$ is positive (which indicates that the reaction is unfavorable at standard conditions)?[9]
- Does K_{eq} indicate the rate at which a reaction will proceed?[10]
- When K_{eq} is large, which has lower free energy: products or reactants?[11]
- When Q is large, which has lower free energy: products or reactants?[12]
- Which direction, forward or backward, will be favored in a reaction if $\Delta G = 0$? (*Hint*: What does Equation 4 look like when $\Delta G = 0$?)[13]
- Radiolabeled chemicals are often used to trace constituents in biochemical reactions. The following reaction with $\Delta G = 0$ is in aqueous solution:

$$A \rightleftharpoons B + C, \quad K_{eq} = \frac{[B][C]}{[A]}$$

A small amount of radiolabeled B is added to the solution. After a period of time, where will the radiolabel most likely be found: in A, in B, or in both?[14]

In summary, then, there are two factors that determine whether a reaction will occur spontaneously (ΔG negative) in the cell:

1) The intrinsic properties of the reactants and products (K_{eq})
2) The concentrations of reactants and products ($RT \ln Q$)

(In the lab there is third factor: temperature. If $\ln Q$ is negative and the temperature is high enough, ΔG will be negative, regardless of the value of $\Delta G^{\circ\prime}$.)

---

[9] The reaction may be favorable ($\Delta G < 0$) if the ratio of the concentrations of reactants to products is sufficiently large to drive the reaction forward (that is, if RT ln Q is more negative than $\Delta G^{\circ\prime}$ is positive, which would make their sum (which, by Equation 4, is ΔG) negative).

[10] K_{eq} indicates only the relative concentrations of reagents once equilibrium is reached, not the reaction rate (how fast equilibrium is reached).

[11] A large K_{eq} means that more products are present at equilibrium. Remember that equilibrium tends toward the lowest energy state. Hence, when K_{eq} is large, products have lower free energy than reactants.

[12] The size of Q says nothing about the properties of the reactants and products. Q is calculated from whatever the initial concentrations happen to be. It is K_{eq} that says something about the nature of reactants and products, since it describes their concentrations after equilibrium has been reached.

[13] If ΔG is 0, then neither the forward nor the reverse reaction is favored. Look at Equations 3 and 4. Note that when $\Delta G = 0$, Equation 4 reduces to Equation 3, and thus $Q = K_{eq}$ (which means Q at this moment is the same as K_{eq}, measured after the reaction system is allowed to reach equilibrium). When $Q = K_{eq}$, we are by definition at equilibrium. Understand and memorize the following: when $\Delta G = 0$, you are at equilibrium; forward reaction rate equals back reaction rate, and the net concentrations of reactants and products do not change.

[14] The reaction is in dynamic equilibrium where reactions are occurring in both directions, but at an equal rate. Because $\Delta G = 0$, we know that the forward reaction and the reverse reaction proceed at equal rates, even though we don't know the actual value. Therefore, after a period of time, the radiolabel will be present in both A and B.

Thermodynamics vs. Reaction Rates

The term *spontaneous* is used to describe a reaction system with $\Delta G < 0$. This can be misleading, since the common usage of the word *spontaneous* has a connotation of *rapid rate*; this is not what spontaneous means in the context of chemical reactions. For example, many reactions have a negative ΔG, indicating that they are "spontaneous" from a thermodynamic point of view, but they do not necessarily occur at a significant rate. Spontaneous means that a reaction is energetically favorable, *but it says nothing about the rate of reaction.*

Thermodynamics will tell you where a system starts and finishes but nothing about the path traveled to get there. The difference in free energy in a reaction is only a function of the nature of the reactants and products. Thus, ΔG does not depend on the pathway a reaction takes or the rate of reaction; it is only a measurement of the difference in free energy between reactants and products.

3.2   KINETICS AND ACTIVATION ENERGY (E_A)

The reason some spontaneous (i.e., *thermodynamically favorable*) reactions proceed very slowly or not at all is that a large amount of energy is required to get them going. For example, the burning of wood is spontaneous, but you can stare at a log all day and it won't burn. Some energy (heat) must be provided to kick-start the process.

The study of reaction rates is called **chemical kinetics**. All reactions proceed through a **transition state (TS)** that is unstable and takes a great deal of energy to produce. The transition state exists for a very, very short time, either moving forward to form products or breaking back down into reactants. The energy required to produce the transition state is called the **activation energy** (E_a). This is the barrier that prevents many reactions from proceeding even though the ΔG for the reaction may be negative. The match you use to light your fireplace provides the activation energy for the reaction known as burning. It is the activation energy barrier that determines the kinetics of a reaction. [How would the rate of a spontaneous reaction be affected if the activation energy were lowered?[15]]

The concept of E_a is key to understanding the role of enzymes, so let's spend some time on it. To illustrate, take this reaction:

$$\text{Bob}_{\text{without a job}} + \text{job} \rightarrow \text{Bob}_{\text{with a job}}$$

Is this a favorable reaction, i.e., will the universe be better off, with less total (nervous) energy, if Bob gets the job? Will things settle down? Let's assume yes. However, between the two states (without/with), there is a temporary state, namely, $\text{Bob}_{\text{applying for job}}$. So the reaction will look this way:

$$\text{Bob}_{\text{without a job}} + \text{job} \rightarrow [\text{Bob}_{\text{applying for job}}]^{\ddagger} \rightarrow \text{Bob}_{\text{with a job}}$$

---

[15] The rate would be increased, since lowering E_a is tantamount to reducing the energy required to achieve the transition state. The more transition state products that are formed, the greater the amount of product produced, i.e., the more rapid the rate of reaction.

The middle term is the transition state, traditionally written in square brackets with a double-cross symbol: [TS]‡. The energy required for Bob to be job hunting is much higher than the energy of Bob with a job *or* Bob without a job. As a result, he may not go job hunting, even though he'd be happier in the long run if he did. In this model, we can describe the E_a as the energy necessary to get Bob to apply for a job.

A **catalyst** lowers the E_a of a reaction *without changing the* ΔG. The catalyst lowers the E_a by *stabilizing the transition state*, making its existence less thermodynamically unfavorable. The second important characteristic of a catalyst is that it is not consumed in the reaction; it is *regenerated* with each reaction cycle.

In our model, an example of a catalyst would be a career planning service (CPS). Adding a CPS won't make Bob$_{without\ a\ job}$ any happier or sadder, nor will it make Bob$_{with\ a\ job}$ happier or sadder. But it will make it much easier for Bob to move between the two states: without a job versus with a job. The traditional way to represent a reaction system like this is using a *reaction coordinate* graph, as shown in Figure 1. This is just a way to look at the energy of the reaction system as compared to the three possible states of the system: 1) reactants, 2) [TS]‡, and 3) products. The *x*-axis plots the physical progress of the reaction system (the "reaction coordinate"), and the *y*-axis plots energy.

Figure 1   The Reaction Coordinate Graph

Enzymes are biological catalysts. They increase the rate of a reaction by lowering the reaction's activation energy, but they *do not affect* ΔG between reactants and products. As catalysts, enzymes have a kinetic role, *not* a thermodynamic one. [Will an enzyme alter the concentration of reagents at equilibrium?[16]] Enzymes may alter the rate of a reaction enormously: a reaction that would take a hundred years to reach equilibrium without an enzyme may occur in just seconds with an enzyme. More information on enzymes can be found in Chapter 4.

---

[16] No. It will affect only the rate at which the reactants and products reach equilibrium.

3.3 OXIDATION AND REDUCTION

Energy Metabolism and the Definitions of Oxidation and Reduction

Where does the energy in foods come from? How do we make use of this energy? Why do we breathe? The answers begin with **photosynthesis**, the process by which plants store energy from the sun in the bond energy of carbohydrates. Plants are **photoautotrophs** because they use energy from light ("photo") to make their own ("auto") food. We are **chemoheterotrophs**, because we use the energy of chemicals ("chemo") produced by other ("hetero") living things, namely plants and other animals. Plants and animals store chemical energy in reduced molecules such as carbohydrates and fats. These reduced molecules are oxidized to produce CO_2 and ATP. The energy of ATP is used in turn to drive the energetically unfavorable reactions of the cell. That's the basic energetics of life; all the rest is detail.

In essence, the production and utilization of energy boil down to a series of oxidation/reduction reactions. **Oxidation** is a chemical term meaning the loss of electrons. **Reduction** means the opposite, the gain of electrons. Molecules can gain or lose electrons depending on the other atoms that they are bound to. There are three common ways to identify oxidation/reduction reactions on the MCAT, and it is important for you to know them:

Recognizing Oxidation Reactions:

1) gain of oxygen atoms
2) loss of hydrogen atoms
3) loss of electrons

Recognizing Reduction Reactions (just the opposite):

1) loss of oxygen atoms
2) gain of hydrogen atoms
3) gain of electrons

Though you should memorize this, it is not a subject worthy of philosophizing. If you can answer questions like the following, you're set: is changing CH_3CH_3 to $H_2C=CH_2$ an oxidation, a reduction, or neither?[17] What about changing Fe^{3+} to Fe^{2+}?[18] What about this: $O_2 \rightarrow H_2O$?[19] You can also identify oxidation/reduction reactions visually by looking at the structure of the molecules. Is the formation of a disulfide bond (Figure 2) an oxidation or a reduction reaction?[20]

---

[17] It's an oxidation, because hydrogens have been removed.

[18] It's a reduction, because an electron has been added.

[19] It's a reduction, because hydrogens have been added to the oxygen molecule.

[20] It's an oxidation, because hydrogens have been removed.

Figure 2 Formation of a Disulfide Bond

Here is one other important fact about oxidation and reduction: when one atom gets reduced, another one *must* be oxidized; hence the term ***redox pair***. As you study the process of glucose oxidation, you will see that each time an oxidation reaction occurs, a reduction reaction occurs too.

Catabolism is the process of breaking down molecules. The opposite is **anabolism**, which is "building-up" metabolism.[21] For example, the way we extract energy from glucose is by **oxidative catabolism**. We break down the glucose by oxidizing it. The stoichiometry of glucose oxidation looks like this:

$$C_6H_{12}O_6 + 6\,O_2 \rightarrow 6\,CO_2 + 6\,H_2O$$

- What are the two members of the redox pair in this reaction?[22]

As we oxidize foods, we release the stored energy plants received from the sun. But we don't make use of that energy right away. Instead, we store it in the form of ATP. Alternatively, we can use the energy in ATP to generate storage molecules such as glycogen and fatty acids. Fatty acids are generated by successive reductions of a carbon chain, thus anabolic processes are generally reductive.

---

[21] The mnemonics are *cata* = breakdown, as in catastrophe, and *ana* = buildup, sounds like "add-a." (Think of anabolic steroids, which weight-lifters use to bulk up.)

[22] The carbons in the sugar are oxidized (to CO_2), and oxygen is reduced (to H_2O).

3.4   ACIDS AND BASES

There are two important definitions of acids and bases you should be familiar with for biochemistry on the MCAT.

Brønsted-Lowry Acids and Bases

Brønsted and Lowry offered the following definitions:

> *Acids are proton (H^+) donors.*
> *Bases are proton (H^+) acceptors.*

While the often seen hydroxide ions qualify as Brønsted-Lowry bases, many other compounds fit this definition as well. Since a Brønsted-Lowry base is any substance that is capable of accepting a proton, any anion or any neutral species with a lone pair of electrons can function as a base.

If we consider the reversible reaction below:

$$H_2CO_3 + H_2O \rightleftharpoons H_3O^+ + HCO_3^-$$

then according to the Brønsted-Lowry definition, H_2CO_3 and H_3O^+ are acids and HCO_3^- and H_2O are bases. The Brønsted-Lowry definition of acids and bases is the most important one for the MCAT.

Lewis Acids and Bases

Lewis's definitions of acids and bases are broader:

> *Lewis acids are electron-pair acceptors.*
> *Lewis bases are electron-pair donors.*

If we consider the reversible reaction below:

$$AlCl_3 + H_2O \rightleftharpoons (AlCl_3OH)^- + H^+$$

then according to the Lewis definition, $AlCl_3$ and H^+ are acids because they accept electron pairs; H_2O and $(AlCl_3OH)^-$ are bases because they donate electron pairs. Lewis acid/base reactions frequently result in the formation of coordinate covalent bonds. For example, in the reaction above, water acts as a Lewis base, since it donates both of the electrons involved in the coordinate covalent bond between OH^- and $AlCl_3$. $AlCl_3$ acts as a Lewis acid, since it accepts the electrons involved in this bond.

The binding of an oxygen molecule to the iron atom in a heme group is a great biological example of a coordinate covalent bond formed between a Lewis acid and base:

Figure 3 Example of a Coordinate Covalent Bond

- Is oxygen the Lewis acid or Lewis base in the heme group?[23]

Conjugate Acids and Bases

When a Brønsted-Lowry acid donates an H$^+$, the remaining structure is called the **conjugate base** of the acid. Likewise, when a Brønsted-Lowry base bonds with an H$^+$ in solution, this new species is called the **conjugate acid** of the base. To illustrate these definitions, consider this reaction:

$$\text{acid–base conjugates}$$
$$NH_3 + H_2O \quad \rightleftharpoons \quad NH_4^+ + OH^-$$
$$\text{acid–base conjugates}$$

---

[23] Oxygen is donating a pair of electrons to the Fe^{2+} ion and is therefore the Lewis base.

Considering only the forward direction, NH_3 is the base and H_2O is the acid. The products are the conjugate acid and conjugate base of the reactants: NH_4^+ is the conjugate acid of NH_3, and OH^- is the conjugate base of H_2O:

$$\begin{array}{ccc} & \text{acid} \dashrightarrow & \overset{\text{conjugate}}{\text{base}} \\ NH_3 + H_2O & \rightleftharpoons & NH_4^+ + OH^- \\ & \underset{\text{base} \dashrightarrow}{\text{conjugate}} & \text{acid} \end{array}$$

Now consider the reverse reaction in which NH_4^+ is the acid and OH^- is the base. The conjugates are the same as for the forward reaction: NH_3 is the conjugate base of NH_4^+, and H_2O is the conjugate acid of OH^-:

$$\begin{array}{ccc} \overset{\text{conjugate}}{\text{base}} \dashleftarrow & \text{acid} \\ NH_3 + H_2O & \rightleftharpoons & NH_4^+ + OH^- \\ \underset{\text{acid}}{\text{conjugate}} \dashleftarrow & \text{base} \end{array}$$

The difference between a Brønsted-Lowry acid and its conjugate base is that the base is missing an H^+. The difference between a Brønsted-Lowry base and its conjugate acid is that the acid has an extra H^+.

forming conjugates:

$$\text{acid} \underset{+\,H^+}{\overset{-\,H^+}{\rightleftharpoons}} \text{base}$$

The Strengths of Acids and Bases

If we use HA to denote a generic acid, its dissociation in water has the form

$$HA(aq) + H_2O(l) \rightleftharpoons H_3O^+(aq) + A^-(aq)$$

The strength of the acid is directly related to how much the products are favored over the reactants. The equilibrium expression for this reaction is

$$K_a = \frac{[H_3O^+][A^-]}{[HA]}$$

This is written as K_a, rather than K_{eq}, to emphasize that this is the equilibrium expression for an acid-dissociation reaction. In fact, K_a is known as the **acid-ionization** (or **acid-dissociation**) **constant** of the acid (HA). We can rank the relative strengths of acids by comparing their K_a values: the larger the K_a value, the stronger the acid; the smaller the K_a value, the weaker the acid.

- Of the following acids, which one would dissociate to the greatest extent (in water)?[24]
    A) HCN (hydrocyanic acid), $K_a = 6.2 \times 10^{-10}$
    B) HNCO (cyanic acid), $K_a = 3.3 \times 10^{-4}$
    C) HClO (hypochlorous acid), $K_a = 2.9 \times 10^{-8}$
    D) HBrO (hypobromous acid), $K_a = 2.2 \times 10^{-9}$

We can apply the same ideas as above to identify the strength of *bases*. If we use B to denote a generic base, its dissolution in water has the form

$$B(aq) + H_2O(l) \rightleftharpoons HB^+(aq) + OH^-(aq)$$

Similar to acids, the strength of the base is directly related to how much the products are favored over the reactants. If we write the equilibrium constant for this reaction, we get:

$$K_b = \frac{[HB^+][OH^-]}{[B]}$$

This is written as K_b, rather than K_{eq}, to emphasize that this is the equilibrium expression for a base-dissociation reaction. In fact, K_b is known as the **base-ionization** (or **base-dissociation**) **constant**. We can rank the relative strengths of bases by comparing their K_b values: the larger the K_b value, the stronger the base; the smaller the K_b value, the weaker the base.

Amphoteric Substances

Take a look at the dissociation of carbonic acid (H_2CO_3), a weak acid:

$$H_2CO_3(aq) + H_2O(l) \rightleftharpoons H_3O^+(aq) + HCO_3^-(aq) \quad (K_a = 4.5 \times 10^{-7})$$

The conjugate base of carbonic acid is HCO_3^-, which also has an ionizable proton. Carbonic acid is said to be **polyprotic**, because it has more than one proton to donate.

---

[24] **B.** The acid that would dissociate to the greatest extent would have the greatest K_a value. Of the choices given, HNCO (choice B) has the greatest K_a value.

Let's look at how the conjugate base of carbonic acid dissociates:

$$HCO_3^-(aq) + H_2O(l) \rightleftharpoons H_3O^+(aq) + CO_3^{2-}(aq) \quad (K_a = 4.8 \times 10^{-11})$$

In the first reaction, HCO_3^- acts as a base, but in the second reaction, it acts as an acid. Whenever a substance can act as either an acid or a base, we say that it is **amphoteric**. The conjugate base of a weak polyprotic acid is always amphoteric, because it can either donate or accept another proton. Also notice that HCO_3^- is a weaker acid than H_2CO_3; in general, every time a polyprotic acid donates a proton, the resulting species will be a weaker acid than its predecessor. Amino acids, which will be discussed in more detail in the next chapter, are all also amphoteric compounds and very important for the MCAT.

pH

The pH scale measures the concentration of H^+ (or H_3O^+) ions in a solution. Because the molarity of H^+ tends to be quite small and can vary over many orders of magnitude, the pH scale is logarithmic:

$$pH = -\log[H^+]$$

This formula implies that $[H^+] = 10^{-pH}$. Since $[H^+] = 10^{-7} M$ in pure water, the pH of water is 7. At 25°C, this defines a pH neutral solution. If $[H^+]$ is greater than $10^{-7} M$, then the pH will be less than 7, and the solution is said to be acidic. If $[H^+]$ is less than $10^{-7} M$, the pH will be greater than 7, and the solution is basic (or alkaline). Notice that a *low* pH means a *high* $[H^+]$ and the solution is *acidic*; a *high* pH means a *low* $[H^+]$ and the solution is basic.

pH > 7	basic solution
pH = 7	neutral solution
pH < 7	acidic solution

The range of the pH scale for most solutions falls between 0 and 14, but some strong acids and bases extend the scale past this range. For example, a 10 M solution of HCl will fully dissociate into H^+ and Cl^-. Therefore, the $[H^+] = 10 M$, and the pH = –1.

An alternate measurement expresses the acidity or basicity in terms of the hydroxide ion concentration, $[OH^-]$, by using pOH. The same formula applies for hydroxide ions as for hydrogen ions.

$$pOH = -\log[OH^-]$$

This formula implies that $[OH^-] = 10^{-pOH}$.

Acids and bases are inversely related: the greater the concentration of H^+ ions, the lower the concentration of OH^- ions, and vice versa. Since $[H^+][OH^-] = 10^{-14}$ at 25°C, the values of pH and pOH satisfy a special relationship at 25°C:

$$pH + pOH = 14$$

So, if you know the pOH of a solution, you can find the pH, and vice versa. For example, if the pH of a solution is 5, then the pOH must be 9. If the pOH of a solution is 2, then the pH must be 12.

Relationships Between Conjugates

pK_a and pK_b

The definitions of pH and pOH both involve a negative logarithm. In general, "p" of something is equal to the –log of that something. Therefore, the following definitions won't be surprising:

$$pK_a = -\log K_a$$

$$pK_b = -\log K_b$$

Because H^+ concentrations are generally very small and can vary over such a wide range, the pH scale gives us more convenient numbers to work with. The same is true for pK_a and pK_b. Remember that the larger the K_a value, the stronger the acid. Since "p" means "take the negative log of...," the *lower* the pK_a value, the stronger the acid. For example, lactic acid has a K_a of 1.3×10^{-4}, and uric acid has a K_a of 2.5×10^{-6}. Since the K_a of lactic acid is larger than that of uric acid, more molecules of lactic acid than uric acid will dissociate into ions in aqueous solution. In other words, lactic acid is stronger than uric acid. The pK_a of lactic acid is 3.9, and the pK_a of uric acid is 5.6. **The acid with the lower pK_a value is the stronger acid. The same logic applies to pK_b: the lower the pK_b value, the stronger the base.** Memorize this!

- Of the following liquids, which one contains the lowest concentration of H_3O^+ ions?[25]
    - A) Lemon juice (pH = 2.3)
    - B) Blood (pH = 7.4)
    - C) Seawater (pH = 8.5)
    - D) Coffee (pH = 5.1)

- Which of the following compounds is the least acidic?[26]
    - A) CH_3COOH, acetic acid (pK_a = 4.76)
    - B) H_2CO_3, carbonic acid (pK_a = 6.35)
    - C) H_3PO_4, phosphoric acid (pK_a = 2.15)
    - D) HCO_3^-, bicarbonate (pK_a = 10.33)

---

[25] **C.** Since pH = – log [H_3O^+], we know that [H_3O^+] = 1/10 pH. This fraction is smallest when the pH is greatest. Of the choices given, seawater has the highest pH.

[26] **D.** The compound with the highest pK_a is the least acidic. Bicarbonate has the highest pK_a of all the answer choices.

Buffer Solutions

A **buffer** is a solution that resists changing pH when a small amount of acid or base is added. The buffering capacity comes from the presence of a weak acid and its conjugate base (or a weak base and its conjugate acid) in roughly equal concentrations.

Buffers are extremely important because nearly every biological process in the human body is pH-dependent. The H^+ ion commonly functions as a reactant, product, or catalyst in chemical reactions in metabolic pathways. In addition, there are many sources of acids and bases in the body that can cause significant changes in the pH if it weren't for our buffer systems.

The most important buffer system in our blood plasma (and for the MCAT) is the bicarbonate buffer system. This buffer consists of carbonic acid (H_2CO_3) and its conjugate base, bicarbonate (HCO_3^-):

Reaction 1 $\quad\quad H_2CO_3 \rightarrow H^+ + HCO_3^-$

This buffer system is particularly complex because of how carbonic acid is formed in the body. During cellular respiration, an activity that is constantly occurring in our body, our cells produce carbon dioxide (CO_2) as a byproduct. The carbon dioxide can then react in a reversible fashion with water to form carbonic acid:

Reaction 2 $\quad\quad CO_2 + H_2O \rightarrow H_2CO_3$

To understand how this buffer system works, we can consider the following scenario. Let's say you go on a run, causing your muscle tissue to produce lactic acid. The lactic acid would seek to increase the concentration of H^+ ions in your body and thus decrease the pH. As discussed earlier, a drop in pH is problematic; it can severely impact our metabolic processes. However, when the lactic acid produces H^+ ions, Reaction 1 shifts to the left by Le Châtelier's principle, reducing the amount of free H^+ ions. While this shift does not completely prevent the pH from falling, it significantly reduces the degree to which the pH falls.

Chapter 3 Summary

- ΔG, the Gibbs free energy, is the amount of energy in a reaction available to do chemical work.

- For a reaction under any set of conditions, $\Delta G = \Delta H - T\Delta S$.

- If $\Delta G < 0$, the reaction is spontaneous in the forward direction. If $\Delta G > 0$, the reaction is nonspontaneous in the forward direction. If $\Delta G = 0$, the reaction is at equilibrium.

- Kinetics is the study of how quickly a reaction occurs, but it does not determine *whether or not* a reaction will occur.

- Activation energy (E_a) is the minimum energy required to start a reaction and decreases in the presence of a catalyst, thereby increasing the reaction rate.

- Acids are proton donors and electron acceptors; bases are proton acceptors and electron donors.

- The higher the K_a (lower the pK_a), the stronger the acid. The higher the K_b (lower the pK_b), the stronger the base.

- Amphoteric substances may act as either acids or bases.

- $pH = -\log[H^+]$. For a concentration of H^+ given in a 10^{-x} M notation, simply take the negative exponent to find the pH. The same is true for the relationship between $[OH^-]$ and pOH, K_a and pK_a, and K_b and pK_b.

- Buffers resist pH change upon the addition of a small amount of acid or base. The key buffer system in the body is the bicarbonate buffer system.

CHAPTER 3 FREESTANDING PRACTICE QUESTIONS

1. Which of the following best describes the function of enzymes?

A) By decreasing the E_a, enzymes increase both the reaction rate and the total amount of product formed.
B) By making the ΔG of the reaction more negative, enzymes increase the amount of product formed per unit time.
C) By decreasing the energy of the transition state, enzymes increase the amount of product formed per unit time.
D) By making the ΔG of the reaction more positive, enzymes increase the total amount of product formed.

2. Malate dehydrogenase is a key enzyme in TCA cycle, which catalyzes the following reaction, which is unfavorable under standard conditions:

$$C_4H_6O_5 + NAD^+ \rightarrow C_4H_4O_5 + NADH + H^+$$

Which of the following corresponds to the compound that is most likely to be oxidized under standard conditions?

A) $C_4H_6O_5$
B) NAD^+
C) $C_4H_4O_5$
D) NADH

3. All of the following are examples of oxidation-reduction reactions EXCEPT:

I. $C_3H_7O_6P + NAD^+ + P_i \rightarrow C_3H_8O_{10}P_2 + NADH + H^+$
II. $C_6H_{12}O_6 + 6\ O_2 \rightarrow 6\ CO_2 + 6\ H_2O$
III. $C_6H_{14}O_{12}P_2 \rightarrow 2\ C_3H_7O_6P$

A) II only
B) III only
C) I and II only
D) I and III only

4. An acidic Glu residue in a protein (neutral in its protonated form) has a pK_a value of 2.3 in the wild-type protein and is found near a neutral Ile residue. What will be the effect on the pK_a of the Glu residue if a mutation substitutes a positively charged Lys residue for the Ile residue?

A) The pK_a will decrease due to favorable ionic interactions between the deprotonated Glu and Lys residues.
B) The pK_a will decrease due to unfavorable ionic interactions between the deprotonated Glu and Lys residues.
C) The pK_a will increase due to favorable ionic interactions between the deprotonated Glu and Lys residues.
D) The pK_a will increase due to unfavorable ionic interactions between the deprotonated Glu and Lys residues.

5. Which of the following best orders the relative basicity of the side chains of Glu ($pK_a = 4.1$), Cys ($pK_a = 8.3$), and Lys ($pK_a = 10.8$)?

A) Cys > Glu > Lys
B) Lys > Glu > Cys
C) Lys > Cys > Glu
D) Glu > Cys > Lys

6. The cells in your body are constantly undergoing cellular respiration, producing CO_2 as a byproduct. What would happen to the pH of your blood if you were to hold your breath?

A) It would increase.
B) It would be the same.
C) It would decrease.
D) It cannot be determined with the information provided.

CHAPTER 3 PRACTICE PASSAGE

The complexity of hemoglobin's function is exemplified by its chemical structure. Multiple factors are believed to affect the kinetics of oxygen binding to the molecule's active sites. It has been proposed that the binding of oxygen (Figure 1) reduces strain on the heme protein superstructure by counterbalancing the pull of the proximal imidazole. Similarly, increasing basicity of the proximal imidazole (e.g., through loss of a hydrogen atom) is believed to exert additional strain on the heme protein in the deoxygenated state by inducing a dome-shaped molecular structure. Because the binding of oxygen relieves this strain, increasing basicity of the proximal imidazole increases the affinity of the heme for oxygen. The hydrophobic pocket created by hydrocarbon-like residues from adjacent heme proteins are also believed to facilitate oxygenation, though it has been proposed steric hindrance may provide an antagonistic effect. The distal imidazole shown below may inhibit dissociation by stabilizing the oxygen molecule in place.

Figure 1   Summary schematic of selected stereoelectronic factors in oxygen affinity of heme

The net effect of these and other factors affecting oxygen dissociation from hemoglobin can be expressed kinetically:

Equation 1 $\text{Heme} + O_2 \underset{k}{\overset{k'}{\rightleftharpoons}} \text{Heme-}O_2$

A single heme molecule will associate with O_2 to form a heme-O_2 complex with rate constant k'; in a reverse reaction, oxygen will dissociate from the heme-O_2 complex with rate constant k. One study examined the kinetics of association of oxygen at different oxygen-bound states as well as the

implied equilibrium constants (K_{O_2}) for each stage of oxygen association (Table 1).

Heme	k' $(M^{-1} \text{ sec}^{-1} \times 10^{-7})$	k (sec^{-1})	K'_{O_2} $(M^{-1} \times 10^{-6})$
Hb	0.20	1079	0.0019
Hb(O$_2$)	0.39	245	0.016
Hb(O$_2$)$_2$	0.35	30	0.12
Hb(O$_2$)$_3$	4.00	47	0.85

Table 1   Kinetic data pertaining to oxygen association with hemoglobin

Another study examined the thermodynamics of the association of hemoglobin dimers ($\alpha\beta$) to form the tetrameric hemoglobin protein.

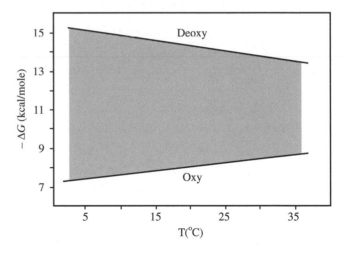

Figure 2   Free energy coupling for dimer-tetramer association in deoxygenated and oxygenated hemoglobin

Extrapolating from the respective linear models depicted in Figure 2, specific data for free energy as well as enthalpy and entropy at body temperature (310 K) are shown in Table 2.

Ligation state	Enthalpy ΔH (kcal/mol)	ΔS (cal/mol-K)	ΔG (kcal/mol)
Oxygenated	4.0	40	−8.4
Deoxygenated	−29.0	−50.1	−−13.5

Table 2   Thermodynamic parameters for dimer-tetramer association of hemoglobin at 310 K

Adapted from Chang, C. K., and Traylor, T. G. *Kinetics of oxygen and carbon monoxide binding to synthetic analogs of the myoglobin and hemoglobin active sites;* Ip, S. H. C., and Ackers, G. K. *Thermodynamic studies on subunit assembly in human hemoglobin.*

1. Based on information presented in the passage, which of the following most likely describes the outcome of replacing the distal imidazole with a nonpolar amino acid residue?

A) The bond between iron and oxygen would be stabilized, decreasing the rate at which oxygen dissociates from hemoglobin.
B) The bond between iron and oxygen would be stabilized, increasing the rate at which oxygen dissociates from hemoglobin.
C) The bond between iron and oxygen would be destabilized, decreasing the rate at which oxygen dissociates from hemoglobin.
D) The bond between iron and oxygen would be destabilized, increasing the rate at which oxygen dissociates from hemoglobin.

2. What is the most likely effect of the addition of acid to the solution in which hemoglobin is suspended?

A) The structure of deoxyhemoglobin would become relatively less strained, reducing affinity for oxygen.
B) The structure of deoxyhemoglobin would become relatively less strained, increasing affinity for oxygen.
C) The structure of deoxyhemoglobin would become relatively more strained, reducing affinity for oxygen.
D) The structure of deoxyhemoglobin would become relatively more strained, increasing affinity for oxygen.

3. Which of the following would be most likely to bind oxygen the fastest in the pulmonary vasculature?

A) Hb
B) $Hb(O_2)$
C) $Hb(O_2)_2$
D) $Hb(O_2)_3$

4. Thermodynamic data for the formation of the hemoglobin tetramer (i.e., association of hemoglobin dimer subunits) provide insight into the "cooperativity" of hemoglobin binding of oxygen. Which of the following statements is most likely to be true based on information in the passage?

A) The positive ΔH for oxyhemoglobin suggests that tetramer association occurs spontaneously at body temperature.
B) The difference in sign between oxygenated and deoxygenated ΔS values suggests that deoxyhemoglobin may be stabilized by increased hydrophobic interactions in the dimer-dimer contact region.
C) The similarity in magnitude of ΔS values supports the idea that the effect of oxygen on the overall order of hemoglobin is incident only at the fourth oxygen binding event.
D) The relatively lesser magnitude of the negative ΔG suggests that oxyhemoglobin dimers will associate more readily than deoxyhemoglobin.

5. At body temperature, which of the following statements is likely true based on the data shown in Table 2?

A) Formation of the deoxygenated hemoglobin tetramer is favored due to more favorable heat of formation.
B) Formation of the deoxygenated hemoglobin tetramer is favored due to more favorable entropy.
C) Formation of the oxygenated hemoglobin tetramer is favored due to more favorable heat of formation.
D) Formation of the oxygenated hemoglobin tetramer is favored due to more favorable entropy.

SOLUTIONS TO CHAPTER 3 FREESTANDING PRACTICE QUESTIONS

1. **C** Enzymes are biological catalysts that affect the kinetics of biological reactions. By lowering the energy of the transition state, enzymes decrease the E_a of biological reactions and increase the amount of product formed per unit time (choice C is correct). ΔG is a thermodynamic quantity and will be unaffected by the addition of an enzyme (choices B and D are wrong). The total amount of product formed once the reaction has reached equilibrium is determined by thermodynamic factors, whereas the amount of product formed in a given time period is determined by kinetic factors (choice A is wrong).

2. **D** Given that the question stem indicates that the reaction is unfavorable under standard conditions, it is likely to proceed in the reverse direction under standard conditions. NADH loses a hydrogen atom in forming NAD$^+$ in the reverse reaction and is thereby oxidized (choice D is correct). Both $C_4H_6O_5$ and NAD$^+$ are more likely to be the product, rather than the reactant, of this redox reaction under standard conditions (choices A and B are wrong). Because $C_4H_4O_5$ gains hydrogen atoms in generating $C_4H_6O_5$, it is reduced, not oxidized (choice C is wrong).

3. **B** Item I is false: NAD$^+$ gains a hydrogen atom and is reduced to NADH, and $C_3H_7O_6P$ must therefore be oxidized. This is an example of a redox reaction and is therefore not an exception (choices C and D can be eliminated). Item II is false: O_2 is in its standard state, giving it a zero oxidation state. It is reduced to have a –2 oxidation state in the products. The O to H ratio is substantially increased in generating CO_2 from $C_6H_{12}O_6$, which indicates $C_6H_{12}O_6$ has been oxidized. This is an example of a redox reaction and is therefore not an exception (choice A can be eliminated, and choice B is correct). Item III is true: this reaction simply splits $C_6H_{12}O_6$ into two three-carbon molecules, while maintaining the O to H ratio. It is not a redox reaction and is therefore the exception.

4. **A** The substitution of a positively charged lysine for a neutral isoleucine would help stabilize Glu in its deprotonated, negatively-charged state (choices B and D can be eliminated). Because it would be more stable, it is more likely to give up its proton (i.e., it becomes more acidic), and the pK_a would decrease (choice C is wrong, and choice A is correct).

5. **C** pK_a is a measure of acid strength. The lower the pK_a, the more acidic the functional group. The question, however, is asking about basicity. Logically, the more acidic the functional group, the less basic it is. Therefore, the most basic group is the one with the highest pK_a, and the least basic is the one with lowest pK_a. Of the three amino acids, the side chain of Lys has the highest pK_a (choices A and D can be eliminated), and the side chain of Glu has the lowest pK_a (choice B can be eliminated, and choice C is correct).

6. **C** When you hold your breath, the CO_2 concentration in your blood increases. The increase in CO_2 will increase the formation of carbonic acid, H_2CO_3, in your blood, which will decrease the pH (choice C is correct; choices A, B, and D are wrong).

SOLUTIONS TO CHAPTER 3 PRACTICE PASSAGE

1. **D**   In its protonated form, the distal imidazole forms a hydrogen bond with the oxygen molecule, stabilizing its position with respect to the iron. Introducing a nonpolar amino acid residue in place of this imidazole would remove the hydrogen bond, destabilizing the interaction between iron and oxygen (choices A and B are wrong). If the interaction between iron and oxygen is destabilized, this would likely result in an increase in the rate at which oxygen dissociates from heme (choice D is correct, and choice C is wrong).

2. **A**   Increasing the acidity of the buffer in which hemoglobin is suspended would effectively *decrease* the basicity of the proximal imidazole by maximizing the chance that H^+ will remain bound to the five-member ring. As a result, the proximal imidazole would exert less strain on the deoxygenated state of hemoglobin (choices C and D can be eliminated). According to the passage, increased basicity of the proximal imidazole this would increase the affinity of the heme for oxygen; therefore, decreased basicity would decrease the affinity for oxygen (choice B can be eliminated, and choice A is correct). Indeed, while there are numerous effects of increasing acidity (decreasing pH) on the heme molecule, the commonly depicted oxygen dissociation curve below demonstrates a relative decrease in heme affinity for oxygen with increasing acidity; higher pO_2 is required for the same oxyhemoglobin saturation.

3. **D**   Table 1 demonstrates that $Hb(O_2)_3$ has the highest k' (rate constant for association) of all the oxygen-bound states of hemoglobin; thus, it can be said that this state would bind oxygen the fastest (choice D is correct). This conclusion is most consistent with the concept of "cooperativity" in binding oxygen to hemoglobin; up to a total of four oxygen molecules, each act of association with oxygen induces structural changes in the heme protein that result in a tendency to increase the rate at which oxygen binds according to the sigmoidal curve shown above in the answer to question 2. All other less-oxygenated states of hemoglobin bind additional oxygen less quickly than $Hb(O_2)_3$ (choices A, B, and C are wrong).

4. **B** ΔS indicates a change in overall disorder consistent with sign; a positive sign indicates increasing disorder, while a negative ΔS indicates an increase in order. Deoxyhemoglobin, with its negative ΔS, thus experiences an increase in order on tetramer association; one reason for this could be increased hydrophobic interactions at the dimer-dimer contact site (i.e., increased stability; choice B is correct). A positive ΔH value implies that the reaction

is *endothermic*, indicating that it requires investment of energy from the surrounding system in order to proceed; while the negative ΔG value indicates that tetramer association is spontaneous for oxyhemoglobin, the positive ΔH actually "works against" this reaction (choice A is wrong). While the fourth oxygen-binding event may be the most rapid per data in Table 1, it is unlikely that previous oxygen-binding events would have had little effect on the overall order of the molecule. Consistent with the "cooperativity" phenomenon of each of these binding events, it is likely that each binding event increases overall *dis*order of the tetramer association reaction incrementally (choice C is wrong). A more negative ΔG indicates increasing spontaneity of the tetramer association; thus tetramer association occurs more spontaneously for deoxyhemoglobin ($\Delta G = -13.5$) than for oxyhemoglobin ($\Delta G = -8.4$; choice D is wrong).

5. **A**   While formation of both the deoxygenated and oxygenated hemoglobin molecules is favored as indicated by negative Gibbs free energy for both reactions, the formation of the deoxygenated tetramer has a more negative ΔG, meaning that this reaction is favored over the formation of a tetramer from oxygenated dimers (choices C and D can be eliminated). Additionally, considering the calculation of Gibbs free energy ($\Delta G = \Delta H - T\Delta S$), the key driver in this case is the change in enthalpy (ΔH), which is negative for the formation of the deoxygenated tetramer. The negative change in entropy (ΔS) for the deoxygenated tetramer actually works against formation, since a negative ΔS indicates an increase in order (decrease in disorder; choice B can be eliminated, and choice A is correct). Note, however, that the magnitude of this spontaneity-decreasing factor is reduced dramatically by the fact that its units include *cal* (not *kcal*) in the numerator position; thus change in entropy is not the driving factor in the spontaneity of tetramer formation for this question.

Chapter 4
Amino Acids and Proteins

The biological macromolecules are grouped into four classes of molecules that play important roles in cells and in organisms as a whole. All of them are polymers, strings of repeated units (monomers).

This chapter discusses amino acids and proteins from a biological perspective: what they are made of, how they are put together, and what their roles are in the body. These molecules are also discussed in *MCAT Organic Chemistry Review* from an organic chemistry perspective: nomenclature, chirality, etc.

4.1 AMINO ACIDS

Proteins are biological macromolecules that act as enzymes, hormones, receptors, channels, transporters, antibodies, and support structures inside and outside cells. Proteins are composed of 20 different amino acids linked together in polymers. The composition and sequence of amino acids in the polypeptide chain is what makes each protein unique and able to fulfill its special role in the cell. Here, we will start with amino acids, the building blocks of proteins, and work our way up to three-dimensional protein structure and function.

Amino Acid Structure and Nomenclature

Understanding the structure of amino acids is key to understanding both their chemistry and the chemistry of proteins. The generic formula for all 20 amino acids is shown below.

Figure 1 Generic Amino Acid Structure

All 20 amino acids share the same nitrogen-carbon-carbon backbone. The unique feature of each amino acid is its **side chain** (variable R-group), which gives it the physical and chemical properties that distinguish it from the other 19.

Classification of Amino Acids

Each of the 20 amino acids is unique because of its side chain, but many of them are similar in their chemical properties. You should be very familiar with the side chains, and it is important to understand the chemical properties that characterize them, such as their varying *shape, ability to hydrogen bond, and ability to act as acids or bases (which determines their charge at physiological pH).*

As you study the 20 amino acids, do so by organizing them into four broad categories: ACIDIC, BASIC, NONPOLAR, and POLAR amino acids. Each amino acid has a three-letter abbreviation and a one-letter abbreviation, which are both important to know for the MCAT.

Acidic Amino Acids

Aspartic acid and glutamic acid are the only amino acids with carboxylic acid functional groups ($pK_a \approx 4$) in their side chains, thereby making the side chains acidic. Thus, there are three functional groups in these amino acids that may act as acids—the two backbone groups and the R-group. You may hear the terms aspart*ate* and glutam*ate*—these simply refer to the anionic (deprotonated) form of each molecule, which is how these amino acids are observed at physiological pH.

Figure 2   Acidic Amino Acids

Basic Amino Acids

Lysine, arginine, and histidine have basic R-group side chains. The pK_a values for the side chains in these amino acids are 10 for Lys, 12 for Arg, and 6.5 for His. Both Lys and Arg are cationic (protonated) at physiological pH, but histidine is unique in having a side chain with a pK_a close to physiological pH. At pH 7.4, histidine may be either protonated or deprotonated—we put it in the basic category, but it often acts as an acid too. This makes it a readily available proton acceptor or donor, explaining its prevalence at protein active sites. A mnemonic is "His goes both ways." This contrasts with amino acids containing –COOH or –NH_2 side chains, which are *always* anionic ($RCOO^-$) or cationic (RNH_3^+) at physiological pH. [By the way, *histamine* is a small molecule that has to do with allergic responses, itching, inflammation, and other processes. (You've heard of antihistamine drugs, for example.) It is not an amino acid; don't confuse it with *histidine*.]

Figure 3   Basic Amino Acids

Hydrophobic (Nonpolar) Amino Acids

Hydrophobic amino acids have either aliphatic (alkyl) or aromatic side chains. Amino acids with aliphatic side chains include glycine, alanine, valine, leucine, and isoleucine. Amino acids with aromatic side chains include phenylalanine, tryptophan, and tyrosine (though the latter is a polar amino acid). Hydrophobic residues tend to associate with each other rather than with water, and therefore are found on the interior of folded globular proteins, away from water. The larger the hydrophobic group, the greater the hydrophobic force repelling it from water.

GLYCINE
Gly
G

ALANINE
Ala
A

VALINE
Val
V

LEUCINE
Leu
L

ISOLEUCINE
Ile
I

PHENYLALANINE
Phe
F

TRYPTOPHAN
Trp
W

Figure 4 Nonpolar Amino Acids

Polar Amino Acids

These amino acids are characterized by an R-group that is polar enough to form hydrogen bonds with water but which does not act as an acid or base. This means they are hydrophilic and will interact with water whenever possible. The hydroxyl groups of serine, threonine, and tyrosine residues are often modified by the attachment of a phosphate group by a regulatory enzyme called a kinase. The result is a change in structure due to the very hydrophilic phosphate group. This modification is an important means of regulating protein activity. This category also includes the amide derivatives of aspartic acid and glutamic acid, which are named asparagine and glutamine, respectively.

SERINE
Ser   **S**

THREONINE
Thr   **T**

TYROSINE
Tyr   **Y**

ASPARAGINE
Asn   **N**

GLUTAMINE
Gln   **Q**

Figure 5 Polar Amino Acids

Sulfur-Containing Amino Acids

Amino acids with sulfur-containing side chains include cysteine and methionine. Cysteine, which contains a thiol (also called a sulfhydryl—like an alcohol that has an S atom instead of an O atom), is fairly polar, and methionine, which contains a thioether (like an ether that has an S atom instead of an O atom), is fairly nonpolar.

CYSTEINE
Cys   **C**

METHIONINE
Met   **M**

Figure 6 Sulfur-Containing Amino Acids

Proline

Proline is unique among the amino acids in that its amino group is covalently bound to its nonpolar side chain, creating a secondary α-amino group and a distinctive ring structure. This unique feature of proline has important consequences for protein folding (see Section 4.3).

PROLINE **P**
Pro

	Hydrophilic		Hydrophobic
ACIDIC	BASIC	POLAR	NONPOLAR
Aspartic acid	Lysine*	Serine	Glycine
Glutamic acid	Arginine	Cysteine	Alanine
	Histidine*	Tyrosine	Valine*
		Threonine*	Leucine*
		Asparagine	Isoleucine*
		Glutamine	Phenylalanine*
			Tryptophan*
			Methionine*
			Proline

*Denotes one of the **nine essential** amino acids, those that cannot be synthesized by adult humans and must be obtained from the diet.

Table 1   Summary Table of Amino Acids

- Which of the following amino acids is most likely to be found on the exterior of a protein at pH 7.0?[1]
  - A) Leucine
  - B) Alanine
  - C) Serine
  - D) Isoleucine

---

[1] Leucine, alanine, and isoleucine are all hydrophobic residues more likely to be found on the interior than the exterior of proteins. Serine (choice **C**), which has a hydroxyl group that can hydrogen bond with water, is the correct answer.

4.2 AMINO ACID REACTIVITY

Since amino acids are composed of an acidic group (the carboxylic acid) and a basic group (the amine), we must be sure to understand the acid/base chemistry of amino acids.

Reviewing the Fundamentals of Acid/Base Chemistry

Recall from the previous chapter that amino acids are **amphoteric**, which means that amino acids can act as acids or bases. This should make sense since an amino acid contains the acidic carboxylic acid group and the basic amino group.

Carboxyl groups of amino acids generally have a pK_a of about 2 (stronger acid), while the ammonium groups generally have a pK_a of 9 or 10 (weaker acid).

The mathematical formula that describes the relationship between pH, pK_a, and the position of equilibrium in an acid-base reaction is known as the **Henderson–Hasselbalch** equation:

$$pH = pK_a + \log \frac{[A^-]}{[HA]} = pK_a + \log \frac{[\text{base form}]}{[\text{acid form}]}$$

Given the pH and the pK_a, we can calculate the ratio of the base and acid forms of a compound at equilibrium. You will go through this equation much more thoroughly in *MCAT General Chemistry Review*. Don't worry too much about doing any calculations here; just make sure you memorize the following rules:

- When the pH of the solution is less than the pK_a of an acidic group, the acidic group will mostly be in its protonated form.
- When the pH of the solution is greater than the pK_a of an acidic group, the acidic group will mostly be in its deprotonated form.

- Which functional group of amino acids has a stronger tendency to donate protons: carboxyl groups (pK_a = 2.0) or ammonium groups (pK_a = 9)? Which group will donate protons at the lowest pH?[2]

---

[2] A high pK_a indicates a weak acid. Acids with a low pK_a tend to deprotonate more easily. Therefore, ammonium groups have a stronger tendency to keep their protons, and carboxyl groups will donate protons at the lowest pH (highest [H^+]).

Application of Fundamental Acid/Base Chemistry to Amino Acids

All amino acids contain an amino group that acts as a base and a carboxyl group ($pK_a \approx 2$) that acts as an acid. In its protonated, or acidic, form, the amine is called an **ammonium group**, and it has a pK_a between 9–10. For example:

$$-NH_3^+ \rightleftharpoons -NH_2 + H^+ \qquad\qquad pK_a \approx 9$$

$$-COOH \rightleftharpoons -COO^- + H^+ \qquad\qquad pK_a \approx 2$$

- Assuming a pK_a of 2, will a carboxylate group be protonated or deprotonated at pH 1.0?[3]
- Will the amino group be protonated or deprotonated at pH 1.0?[4]
- Glycine is the simplest amino acid, with only hydrogen as its R-group. Its only functional groups are the backbone groups discussed above (amino and carboxyl). What will be the net charge on a glycine molecule at pH 12?[5]
- At pH 6.0, between the pK_as of the ammonium and carboxyl groups, what will be the net charge on a molecule of glycine?[6]

Figure 7 Important Amino Acid Conjugate Acid/Base Pairs

The Isoelectric Point of Amino Acids

There is a pH for every amino acid at which it has no overall net charge (the positive and negative charges cancel). A molecule with positive and negative charges that balance is referred to as a dipolar ion or **zwitterion**. The pH at which a molecule is uncharged (zwitterionic) is referred to as its **isoelectric point** (pI). "Zwitter" is German for "hybrid," implying that an amino acid at its pI has both (+) and (–) charges.

---

[3] The pH is less than the pK_a here, so protonation wins over dissociation, and the group will be protonated. The correct answer is –COOH.

[4] The pH is much lower than the pK_a for the ammonium group, so the amino group is protonated: NH_3^+.

[5] Since pH 12 represents a very low [H^+], both groups will become deprotonated (COO^- and NH_2), creating a net charge of –1 per glycine molecule.

[6] The carboxyl group will be deprotonated (COO^-) with a charge of –1, and the amino group will be protonated (NH_3^+) with a charge of +1, creating a net charge of 0 per glycine molecule.

It is possible to calculate the pI of an amino acid—in other words, to figure out the pH value at which (+) and (–) charges balance (that's the definition of pI). For a molecule with two functional groups, such as glycine, the calculation is simple: just *average the pK$_a$s of the two functional groups*. The pI of more complex molecules can also be calculated, but the math is complex. For the MCAT, you should know how to calculate the pI of a molecule with two functional groups (with no acidic or basic functional groups in the side chain). Another important thing to know for the MCAT is how to compare the pH of a solution to the pK$_a$ of a functional group of an amino acid and determine if a site is mostly protonated or deprotonated. If the pH is higher than the pK$_a$, the site is mostly deprotonated; if the pH is lower than the pK$_a$, the site is mostly protonated. This can be illustrated in the titration curve (titrations will be discussed in more detail in *MCAT General Chemistry Review*) for glycine:

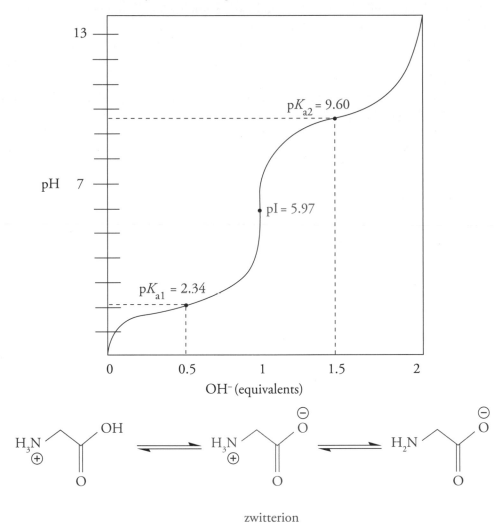

zwitterion

- What is the pI of glycine?[7]

---

[7] To calculate the pI, just average the pK$_a$s of the two functional groups: (9.60 + 2.34)/2 = 5.97, or roughly 6 (this will be discussed in more detail in *MCAT Organic Chemistry Review*).

4.3 PROTEIN STRUCTURE

There are two common types of covalent bonds between amino acids in proteins: the **peptide bonds** that link amino acids together into polypeptide chains and **disulfide bridges** between cysteine R-groups.

The Peptide Bond

Polypeptides are formed by linking amino acids together in peptide bonds. A peptide bond is formed between the carboxyl group of one amino acid and the α-amino group of another amino acid with the loss of water. The figure below shows the formation of a dipeptide from the amino acids glycine and alanine.

Figure 8   Peptide Bond (Amide Bond) Formation

In a polypeptide chain, the N–C–C–N–C–C pattern formed from the amino acids is known as the **backbone** of the polypeptide. An individual amino acid is termed a **residue** when it is part of a polypeptide chain. The amino terminus is the first end made during polypeptide synthesis, and the carboxy terminus is made last. Hence, by convention, the amino-terminal residue is also always written first.

- In the oligopeptide Phe-Glu-Gly-Ser-Ala, state the number of acid and base functional groups, which residue has a free α-amino group, and which residue has a free α-carboxyl group. (Refer to the beginning of the chapter for structures.)[8]
- How many unique dipeptides (made from linking two amino acids) can be synthesized using only alanine and glycine residues?[9]

---

[8] As stated above, the amino end is always written first. Therefore, the oligopeptide begins with an exposed Phe amino group and ends with an exposed Ala carboxyl; all the other backbone groups are hitched together in peptide bonds. Out of all the R-groups, there is only one acidic or basic functional group, the acidic glutamate R-group. This R-group plus the two terminal backbone groups gives a total of three acid/base functional groups.

[9] Four (Gly-Gly, Ala-Ala, Gly-Ala, Ala-Gly). Note that Ala-Gly and Gly-Ala are not identical peptides. In Ala-Gly, the N-terminus is Ala and the C-terminus is Gly. In Gly-Ala, the N-terminus is Gly and the C-terminus is Ala.

- Thermodynamics states that free energy must decrease for a reaction to proceed spontaneously and that such a reaction will spontaneously move toward equilibrium. The diagram below shows the free energy changes during peptide bond formation. At equilibrium, which is thermodynamically favored: the dipeptide or the individual amino acids?[10]

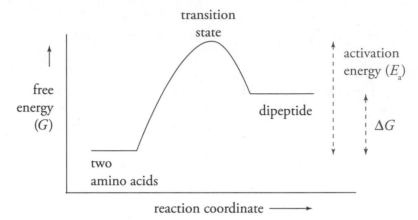

- In that case, how are peptide bonds formed and maintained inside cells?[11]

Hydrolysis of a protein by another protein is called **proteolysis** or **proteolytic cleavage**, and the protein that does the cutting is known as a **proteolytic enzyme** or **protease**. Proteolytic cleavage is a specific means of cleaving peptide bonds. Many enzymes only cleave the peptide bond adjacent to a specific amino acid. For example, the protease trypsin cleaves on the carboxyl side of the positively charged (basic) residues arginine and lysine, while chymotrypsin cleaves adjacent to large hydrophobic residues such as phenylalanine. (Do *not* memorize these examples.)

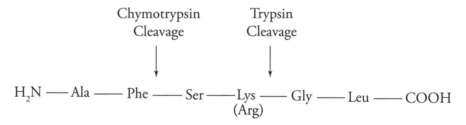

Figure 9   Specificity of Protease Cleavage

- Based on the above, if the following peptide is cleaved by trypsin, what amino acid will be on the new N-terminus and how many fragments will result: Ala-Gly-Glu-Lys-Phe-Phe-Lys?[12]

---

[10] The dipeptide has a higher free energy, so its existence is less favorable. In other words, existence of the chain is less favorable than existence of the isolated amino acids.

[11] During protein synthesis, stored energy is used to force peptide bonds to form. Once the bond is formed, even though its destruction is thermodynamically favorable, it remains stable because the activation energy for the hydrolysis reaction is so high. In other words, hydrolysis is thermodynamically favorable but kinetically slow.

[12] Trypsin will cleave on the carboxyl side of the Lys residue, with Phe on the N-terminus of the new Phe-Phe-Lys fragment. There will be two fragments after trypsin cleavage: Phe-Phe-Lys and Ala-Gly-Glu-Lys.

The Disulfide Bond

Cysteine is an amino acid with a reactive thiol (sulfhydryl, SH) in its side chain. The thiol of one cysteine can react with the thiol of another cysteine to produce a covalent sulfur-sulfur bond known as a disulfide bond, as illustrated below. The cysteines forming a disulfide bond may be located in the same or different polypeptide chain(s). The disulfide bridge plays an important role in stabilizing tertiary protein structure; this will be discussed in the section on protein folding. Once a cysteine residue becomes disulfide-bonded to another cysteine residue, it is called *cystine* instead of cysteine.

Figure 10   Formation of the Disulfide Bond

- Which is more oxidized, the sulfur in *cysteine* or the sulfur in *cystine*?[13]
- The inside of cells is known as a reducing environment because cells possess antioxidants (chemicals that prevent oxidation reactions). Where would disulfide bridges be more likely to be found, in extracellular proteins, under oxidizing conditions, or in the interior of cells, in a reducing environment?[14]

Protein Structure in Three Dimensions

Each protein folds into a unique three-dimensional structure that is required for that protein to function properly. Improperly folded, or **denatured**, proteins are nonfunctional. There are four levels of protein folding that contribute to their final three-dimensional structure. Each level of structure is dependent upon a particular type of bond, as discussed in the following sections.

---

[13] In forming cystine from two cysteine residues, hydrogen atoms are removed (an oxidation reaction), indicating that the sulfur in cystine is more oxidized.

[14] In a reducing environment, the S-S group is reduced to two SH groups. Disulfide bridges are found only in extracellular polypeptides, where they will not be reduced. Examples of protein complexes held together by disulfide bridges include antibodies and the hormone insulin.

Denaturation is an important concept. It refers to the **disruption of a protein's shape without breaking peptide bonds**. Proteins are denatured by *urea* (which disrupts hydrogen bonding interactions), by *extremes of pH*, by extremes of *temperature,* and by *changes in salt concentration (tonicity).*

Primary (1°) Structure: The Amino Acid Sequence

The simplest level of protein structure is the order of amino acids bonded to each other in the polypeptide chain. This linear ordering of amino acid residues is known as primary structure. **Primary structure** is the same as **sequence**. The bond which determines 1° structure is the peptide bond, simply because this is the bond that links one amino acid to the next in a polypeptide.

Secondary (2°) Structure: Hydrogen Bonds Between Backbone Groups

Secondary structure refers to the initial folding of a polypeptide chain into shapes stabilized by hydrogen bonds between backbone NH and CO groups. Certain motifs of secondary structure are found in most proteins. The two most common are the α-**helix** and the β-**pleated sheet**.

All α-helices have the same well-defined dimensions that are depicted below with the R-groups omitted for clarity. The α-helices of proteins are always right-handed, 5 angstroms in width, with each subsequent amino acid rising 1.5 angstroms. There are 3.6 amino acid residues per turn with the α-carboxyl oxygen of one amino acid residue hydrogen-bonded to the α-amino proton of an amino acid three residues away. (*Don't* memorize these numbers, but *do* try to visualize what they mean.)

Figure 11   An α-Helix

The unique side chain of proline causes two problems in polypeptide chains:

1. The formation of a peptide bond with proline (shown below) eliminates the only hydrogen atom on the nitrogen atom of proline. The absence of the N-H bond disrupts the backbone hydrogen bonding in the polypeptide chain.
2. The unique structure of proline forces it to kink the polypeptide chain.

For both reasons, proline residues never appear within the α-helix.

Figure 12 Proline

Proteins such as hormone receptors and ion channels are often found with α-helical transmembrane regions integrated into the hydrophobic membranes of cells. The α-helix is a favorable structure for a hydrophobic transmembrane region because all polar NH and CO groups in the backbone are hydrogen-bonded to each other on the inside of the helix, and thus don't interact with the hydrophobic membrane interior. α-Helical regions that span membranes also have hydrophobic R-groups, which radiate out from the helix, interacting with the hydrophobic interior of the membrane.

β-pleated sheets are also stabilized by hydrogen bonding between NH and CO groups in the polypeptide backbone. In β-sheets, however, hydrogen bonding occurs between residues distant from each other in the chain or even on separate polypeptide chains. Also, the backbone of a β-sheet is extended, rather than coiled, with side groups directed above and below the plane of the β-sheet. There are two types of β-sheets, one with adjacent polypeptide strands running in the *same* direction (**parallel** β-pleated sheet) and another in which the polypeptide strands run in *opposite* directions (**antiparallel** β-pleated sheet).

Figure 13   A β-Pleated Sheet

- If a single polypeptide folds once and forms a β-pleated sheet with itself, would this be a parallel or antiparallel β-pleated sheet?[15]
- What effect would a molecule that disrupts hydrogen bonding, such as urea, have on protein structure?[16]

Tertiary (3°) Structure: Hydrophobic/Hydrophilic Interactions

The next level of protein folding, tertiary structure, concerns interactions between amino acid residues located more distantly from each other in the polypeptide chain. These interactions may include van der Waals forces between nonpolar side chains, hydrogen bonds between polar side chains, disulfide bonds between cysteine residues, and electrostatic interactions between acidic and basic side chains. The folding of secondary structures such as α-helices into higher order tertiary structures is driven by interactions of R-groups with each other and with the solvent (water). Hydrophobic R-groups tend to fold into the interior of the protein, away from the solvent, and hydrophilic R-groups tend to be exposed to water on the surface of the protein (shown for the generic globular protein). This is called the **hydrophobic effect.**

---

[15] It would be antiparallel because one participant in the β-pleated sheet would have a C to N direction, while the other would be running N to C.

[16] Putting a protein in a urea solution will disrupt H-bonding, thus disrupting secondary structure (and possibly tertiary and quaternary) by unfolding α-helices and β-sheets. It would not affect primary structure, which depends on the much more stable peptide bond. Disruption of 2°, 3°, or 4° structure without breaking peptide bonds is *denaturation*.

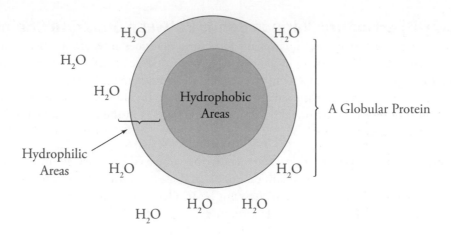

Figure 14 Folding of a Globular Protein in Aqueous Solution

Under the right conditions, the forces driving hydrophobic avoidance of water and hydrogen bonding will fold a polypeptide spontaneously into the correct conformation, the lowest energy conformation. In a classic experiment by Christian Anfinsen and coworkers, the effect of a denaturing agent (urea) and a reducing agent (β-mercaptoethanol) on the folding of a protein called ribonuclease was examined. In the following questions, you will reenact their thought processes. Try to answer the questions before reading the footnotes.

- Ribonuclease has eight cysteines that form four disulfides bonds. What effect would a reducing agent have on its tertiary structure?[17]
- If the disulfides serve only to lock into place a tertiary protein structure that forms first on its own, then what effect would the reducing agent have on correct protein folding?[18]
- Would a protein end up folded normally if you (1) first put it in a reducing environment, (2) then denatured it by adding urea, (3) next removed the reducing agent, allowing disulfide bridges to reform, and (4) finally removed the denaturing agent?[19]
- What if you did the same experiment but in this order: 1, 2, 4, 3?[20]
- Which of the following may be considered an example of tertiary protein structure?[21]
  - I.   van der Waals interactions between two Phe R-groups located far apart on a polypeptide
  - II. Hydrogen bonds between backbone amino and carboxyl groups
  - III. Covalent disulfide bonds between cysteine residues located far apart on a polypeptide

---

[17] The disulfide bridges would be broken. Tertiary structure would be less stable.

[18] The shape should not be disrupted if breaking disulfides is the only disturbance. It's just that the shape would be less sturdy—like a concrete wall without the rebar.

[19] No. If you allow disulfide bridges to form while the protein is still denatured, it will become locked into an abnormal shape.

[20] You should end up with the correct structure. In step 1, you break the reinforcing disulfide bridges. In step 2, you denature the protein completely by disrupting H-bonds. In step 4, you allow the H-bonds to reform; as stated in the text, normally the correct tertiary structure will form spontaneously if you leave the polypeptide alone. In step 3, you reform the disulfide bridges, thus locking the structure into its correct form.

[21] **Item I is true:** this is a good example of 3°. Item II is false: this describes 2°, not 3° structure. **Item III is true:** this describes the disulfide bond, which is another example of tertiary structure.

Quaternary (4°) Structure: Various Bonds Between Separate Chains

The highest level of protein structure, quaternary structure, describes interactions between polypeptide subunits. A **subunit** is a single polypeptide chain that is part of a large complex containing many subunits (a **multisubunit complex**). The arrangement of subunits in a multisubunit complex is what we mean by quaternary structure. For example, mammalian RNA polymerase II contains 12 different subunits. The interactions between subunits are instrumental in protein function, as in the cooperative binding of oxygen by each of the four subunits of hemoglobin.

The forces stabilizing quaternary structure are generally the same as those involved in tertiary structure—van der Waals forces, hydrogen bonds, disulfide bonds, and electrostatic interactions. It is key to understand, however, that there is one bond that may not be involved in quaternary structure—the peptide bond—because this bond defines sequence (1° structure).

- What is the difference between a disulfide bridge involved in quaternary structure and one involved in tertiary structure?[22]

4.4 PROTEINS AS ENZYMES

Enzymes are biological catalysts. They increase the rate of a reaction by lowering the reaction's activation energy, but they *do not affect* ΔG between reactants and products. As catalysts, enzymes have a kinetic role, *not* a thermodynamic one. Enzymes may alter the rate of a reaction enormously: a reaction that would take a hundred years to reach equilibrium without an enzyme may occur in just seconds with an enzyme.

Given that thousands of enzymes have been discovered, scientists frequently classify them based upon reaction type. Table 2 lists several examples but note that enzymes cannot control the direction in which a reaction proceeds; it is common to see enzymes in a given class function in reverse.

Enzyme Class	Reaction
Hydrolase	hydrolyzes chemical bonds (includes ATPases, proteases, and others)
Isomerase	rearranges bonds within a molecule to form an isomer
Ligase	forms a chemical bond (e.g., DNA ligase)
Lyase	breaks chemical bonds by means other than oxidation or hydrolysis (e.g., pyruvate decarboxylase)
Kinase	transfers a phosphate group to a molecule from a high energy carrier, such as ATP (e.g., phosphofructokinase [PFK])
Oxidoreductase	runs redox reactions (includes oxidases, reductases, dehydrogenases, and others)
Polymerase	polymerization (e.g., addition of nucleotides to the leading strand of DNA by DNA polymerase III)
Phosphatase	removes a phosphate group from a molecule
Phosphorylase	transfers a phosphate group to a molecule from inorganic phosphate (e.g., glycogen phosphorylase)
Protease	hydrolyzes peptide bonds (e.g., trypsin, chymotrypsin, pepsin, etc.)

Table 2 Enzyme Classes

[22] Quaternary disulfides are bonds that form between chains that aren't linked by peptide bonds. Tertiary disulfides are bonds that form between residues in the same polypeptide.

ATP as an Energy Source: Reaction Coupling

Enzymes increase the rate of reactions that have a negative ΔG. These reactions would occur on their own without an enzyme (they are spontaneous) but far more slowly than with one. However, there are many reactions in the body that occur which have a positive ΔG. The biosynthesis of macromolecules such as DNA and protein is not spontaneous ($\Delta G > 0$), but clearly these reactions *do* take place (or we wouldn't be here). How can this be? Thermodynamically unfavorable reactions in the cell can be driven forward by **reaction coupling**. In reaction coupling, one very favorable reaction is used to drive an unfavorable one. This is possible because *free energy changes are additive*. [What is the favorable reaction that the cell can use to drive unfavorable reactions?[23]] In the lab, the $\Delta G^{\circ\prime}$ for the hydrolysis of one phosphate group from ATP is -7.3 kcal/mol, so it is a very favorable reaction. In the cell, ΔG is about -12 kcal/mol, so in the cell it is even more favorable. [What's the difference between the situation *in vitro* (lab) under standard conditions and *in vivo* (cell) under nonstandard conditions?[24]]

4.4

How does ATP hydrolysis drive unfavorable reactions? There are many ways. One example is by causing a conformational change in a protein; in this way ATP hydrolysis can be used to power energy-costly events like transmembrane transport. Another example is by transfer of a phosphate group from ATP to a substrate. Take the unfavorable reaction A + B → C. Let's say that Reactant A must proceed through an intermediate, APO_4^{2-}, in order to participate. Let's say $\Delta G = +7$ kcal/mol for the overall reaction. What if the two partial reactions have ΔGs as follows:

$$A + PO_4^{2-} \rightarrow APO_4^{2-} \qquad \Delta G = \quad +2 \text{ kcal/mol}$$

$$\underline{APO_4^{2-} + B \rightarrow C + PO_4^{2-} \qquad \Delta G = \quad +5 \text{ kcal/mol}}$$

$$Total \quad \Delta G = \quad +7 \text{ kcal/mol}$$

These reactions will not proceed because the overall ΔG will be $+7$ kcal/mol. What will be the *overall* ΔG if we *couple* the reaction A + B → C to the hydrolysis of one ATP? All we have to do is add up all the ΔG values, as follows:

$$ATP \rightarrow ADP + PO_4^{2-} \qquad \Delta G = \quad -12 \text{ kcal/mol}$$

$$A + PO_4^{2-} \rightarrow APO_4^{2-} \qquad \Delta G = \quad +2 \text{ kcal/mol}$$

$$\underline{APO_4^{2-} + B \rightarrow C + PO_4^{2-} \qquad \Delta G = \quad +5 \text{ kcal/mol}}$$

$$Total \quad \Delta G = \quad -5 \text{ kcal/mol}$$

Now the overall reaction, shown below, is thermodynamically favorable. We have *coupled* the unfavorable reaction A + B → C to the highly favorable hydrolysis of ATP:

$$A + B + ATP \rightarrow C + ADP + PO_4^{2-} \quad \Delta G = -5 \text{ kcal/mol}$$

---

[23] ATP hydrolysis!

[24] $Q_{(cell)} \neq K_{eq}$. This means that the relative concentrations of ATP and ADP + P_i are not at equilibrium levels in the cell. Actually, $Q_{(cell)} \ll K_{eq}$ because the cell keeps a high concentration of ATP around.

Note that we first stated that the enzyme has only a kinetic role (influencing rate only), not a thermo-dynamic one (determining favorability). Then we went on to discuss reaction coupling, which allows enzymes to promote otherwise unfavorable reactions. There is no contradiction, however. The only dif-ference is viewing reactions in an isolated manner or in the complex series of linked reactions more com-monly found in the body. The same rule applies in either case: ΔG must be negative for either a single reaction or a series of linked reactions to occur spontaneously. In summary:

- One reaction in a test tube—the enzyme is a catalyst with a kinetic role only. It influences the rate of the reaction, but not the outcome.
- Many "real-life" reactions in the cell—enzyme controls outcomes by selectively promoting unfavorable reactions via reaction coupling.

4.5   ENZYME STRUCTURE AND FUNCTION

Most enzymes are proteins that must fold into specific three-dimensional structures to act as catalysts. (Some enzymes are RNA or contain RNA sequences with catalytic activity. Most catalyze their own splic-ing, and the rRNA in ribosomes helps in peptide-bond formation.) An enzyme may consist of a single polypeptide chain or several polypeptide subunits held together in a ____[25] (primary? secondary? etc.) structure. The reason for the importance of folding in enzyme function is the proper formation of the **active site**, the region in an enzyme's three-dimensional structure that is directly involved in catalysis. [What shape are enzymes more likely to have: fibrous/elongated or globular/spherical?[26]] The reactants in an enzyme-catalyzed reaction are called **substrates**. (Products have no special name; they're just "prod-ucts.") What is the role of the active site, that is, how do enzymes work? The **active site model**, com-monly referred to as the "lock and key hypothesis," states that the substrate and active site are perfectly complementary. This differs from the **induced fit model,** which asserts that the substrate and active site differ slightly in structure and that the binding of the substrate induces a conformational change in the enzyme. The induced fit model has gained greater acceptance in recent years, but regardless of the model, enzymes accelerate the rate of a given reaction by helping to *stabilize the transition state*. For example, if a transition state intermediate possesses a transient negative charge, what amino acid residues might be found at the active site to stabilize the transition state?[27] This lowers the activation energy barrier between reactants and products. In our previous example of Bob looking for a job, the use of a career planning service would function as an enzyme by making the process of job hunting easier.

- Is it possible that amino acids located far apart from each other in the primary protein sequence may play a role in the formation of the same active site?[28]
- If, during an enzyme-catalyzed reaction, an intermediate forms in which the substrate is covalently linked to the enzyme via a serine residue, can this occur at any serine residue or must it occur at a specific serine residue?[29]

---

[25] quaternary

[26] Globular. Structural proteins such as collagen tend to be fibrous, but proteins that act as catalysts tend to be roughly spherical to form an active site in a cleft in the sphere.

[27] A positive charge would stabilize the negative charge in the intermediate. Such a charge might be contributed by His, Arg, or Lys. Alterna-tively, the hydrogen of the $-NH_2$ group in glutamine or asparagine could hydrogen bond with the negative charge.

[28] Yes, the amino acids at the active site may be distant from each other in a polypeptide's primary sequence but be near each other in the final folded protein. This is why protein folding is crucial for enzyme function.

[29] It must occur at a particular serine residue which sticks out into the active site.

- Compound A converts into Compound B in solution: $A \rightleftharpoons B$. The reaction has the following equilibrium constant: $K_{eq} = [B]_{eq}/[A]_{eq} = 1{,}000$. If pure A is dissolved in water at 298 K, will ΔG for the reaction $A \rightleftharpoons B$ be positive or negative? Is it possible to answer this question without knowing $\Delta G^{\circ\prime}$?[30]
- Regarding the reaction described in the previous question, if pure B is put into solution in the presence of an enzyme that catalyzes the reaction between A and B, which one of the following will be true?[31]
    - A) All the B will be converted into A, until there is 1,000 times more A than B.
    - B) All of the B will remain as B, since B is favored at equilibrium.
    - C) The enzyme will have no effect, since enzymes act on the transition state and there is no transition state present.
    - D) The reaction that produces A will predominate until $\Delta G = 0$.

4.5

The active site for enzymes is generally highly specific in its substrate recognition, including stereospecificity (the ability to distinguish between stereoisomers). For example, enzymes which catalyze reactions involving amino acids are specific for D or L amino acids, and enzymes catalyzing reactions involving monosaccharides may distinguish between stereoisomers as well. [Which configurations are found in animals?[32]]

Many **proteases** (protein-cleaving enzymes) have an active site with a serine residue whose OH group can act as a nucleophile, attacking the carbonyl carbon of an amino acid residue in a polypeptide chain. Examples are trypsin, chymotrypsin, and elastase. These enzymes also usually have a **recognition pocket** near the active site. This is a pocket in the enzyme's structure which attracts certain residues on substrate polypeptides. The enzyme always cuts polypeptides at the same site, just to one side of the recognition residue. For example, chymotrypsin always cuts on the carboxyl side of one of the large hydrophobic or aromatic residues Tyr, Trp, Phe, and Met. Enzymes that act on hydrophobic substrates have hydrophobic amino acids in their active sites, while hydrophilic/polar amino acids will comprise the active site of enzymes with hydrophilic substrates.

Given the importance of the active site, it becomes clear that small alterations in its structure can drastically alter enzymatic activity. Therefore, both temperature and pH play a critical role in enzymatic function. As temperature increases, the thermal motion of the peptide and surrounding solution destabilize its structure. If the temperature rises sufficiently, the protein **denatures** and loses its orderly structure. The pH of the surrounding medium also impacts protein stability; several amino acids possess ionizable –R groups that change charge depending on pH. This can decrease the affinity of a substrate for the active site and, if the pH deviates sufficiently, the protein can denature.

---

[30] You don't need to calculate $\Delta G^{\circ\prime}$; all you need to know is that with a K_{eq} of 1,000, there will be 1,000 times more B than A in solution at equilibrium. If we create a solution with only A, the reaction must move spontaneously toward B.

[31] If only B exists in solution, then the back-reaction producing A will predominate until equilibrium is reached ($\Delta G = 0$), regardless of the presence or absence of enzyme (choice **D** is correct, and choice B is wrong). According to the K_{eq} given, at equilibrium there will be 1,000 times more B than A, not the other way around (choice A is wrong). Note that enzymes do not act on the transition state; they act to produce the transition state (choice C is wrong).

[32] L amino acids and D sugars. Remember the L in aLanine.

- The transition state for a reaction possesses a transient negative charge. The active site for an enzyme catalyzing this reaction contains a His residue to stabilize the intermediate. If the His residue at the active site is replaced by a glutamate that is negatively charged at pH 7.0, what effect will this have on the reaction, assuming that the reactants are present in excess compared to the enzyme?[33]
    - A) The repulsion caused by the negative charge in the glutamate at the altered active site will increase the activation energy and make the reaction proceed more slowly than it would in a solution without enzyme.
    - B) The rate of catalysis will be unaffected, but the equilibrium ratio of products and reactants will change, favoring reactants.
    - C) The transition state intermediate will not be stabilized as effectively by the altered enzyme, lowering the rate relative to the rate with catalysis by the normal enzyme.
    - D) The rate of catalysis will decrease, and the equilibrium constant will change.

Enzymatic function can also depend upon the association of additional molecules. **Cofactors**, which are metal ions or small molecules (not themselves a protein), are required for activity in many enzymes. In fact, the majority of the vitamins in our diet serve as precursors for cofactors (e.g., niacin [B3] is ultimately transformed into NAD^+). When a cofactor is an organic molecule, it is referred to as a **coenzyme**; these often bind to the substrate during the catalyzed reaction. One prime example of a coenzyme, which we will focus on later in the chapter, is coenzyme A (CoA).

4.6   REGULATION OF ENZYME ACTIVITY

Metabolic pathways in the cell are not all continually on, but must be tightly regulated to maintain health. For example, if glycogen synthesis and breakdown occur in the same cell at the same time, a great deal of energy will be wasted without accomplishing anything. Therefore, the activity of key enzymes in metabolic pathways is usually regulated in one or more of the following ways:

1) **Covalent modification.** Proteins can have several different groups covalently attached to them, and this can regulate their activity, lifespan in the cell, and/or cellular location. The addition of a phosphoryl group from a molecule of ATP by a protein **kinase** to the hydroxyl of serine, threonine, or tyrosine residues is the most common example. Phosphorylation of these different sites on an enzyme can either activate or inactivate the enzyme. Protein **phosphorylases** also phosphorylate proteins, but use free-floating inorganic phosphate (P_i) in the cell instead of ATP. Protein phosphorylation can be reversed by protein **phosphatases**.

2) **Proteolytic cleavage.** Many enzymes (and other proteins) are synthesized in inactive forms (zymogens) that are activated by cleavage by a protease.

---

[33] Beware of long, complex-sounding questions! They may not be as bad as they look; for instance, the phrase "assuming that the reactants are present in excess compared to the enzyme" adds nothing to the substance of this question. If His (which is positive or neutral at pH 7) is replaced by Glu (negatively charged at pH 7), this could decrease the effectiveness of—or destroy altogether—the active site of the enzyme. This means the transition state would not be effectively stabilized, and the rate of the reaction would simply reduce to that of the uncatalyzed reaction (choice **C** is correct). The rate would not proceed more slowly than the uncatalyzed reaction (i.e., "in solution without enzyme"; choice A is wrong), and remember that enzymes do not alter reaction equilibria (K_{eq} will be unaffected; choices B and D are wrong).

3) **Association with other polypeptides.** Some enzymes have catalytic activity in one polypeptide subunit that is regulated by association with a separate regulatory subunit. For example, there are some proteins that demonstrate continuous rapid catalysis if their regulatory subunit is removed; this is known as **constitutive activity** (*constitutive* means continuous or unregulated). There are other proteins that require association with another peptide in order to function. Still other proteins can bind many regulatory subunits. There are numerous examples of this in the cell, and many of them have diverse and complex regulatory mechanisms that all revolve around the theme of "associations with other polypeptides can affect enzyme activity."

4) **Allosteric regulation.** The modification of active-site activity through interactions of molecules with other specific sites on the enzyme (called **allosteric sites**). Let's look at this in a little more detail.

Allosteric Regulation

If the cell is to make use of the enzyme as a biochemical switch, there must be a way to turn the enzyme *on* or *off*. One mechanism of regulation is the binding of small molecules to particular sites on an enzyme that are distinct from the active site; this is allosteric regulation. This name comes from the fact that the particular spot on the enzyme which can bind the small molecule is *not* the active site; *allo* means "other," and *steric* refers to a location in space (as in "steric hindrance"), so *allosteric* means "at another place." The binding of the allosteric regulator to the allosteric site is generally noncovalent and reversible. When bound, the allosteric regulator can alter the conformation of the enzyme to increase or decrease catalysis, even though it may be bound to the enzyme at a site distant from the active site or even on a separate polypeptide.

Feedback Inhibition

Enzymes usually act as part of pathways, not alone. Rather than regulate every enzyme in a pathway, usually there are one or two key enzymes that are regulated, such as the enzyme that catalyzes the first irreversible step in a pathway. The easiest way to explain this is with an example. Three enzymes (E1, E2, and E3) catalyze the three steps required to convert Substrate A to Product D. When plenty of D is around, it would be logical to shut off E1 so that excess B, C, and D are not made. This would conserve A and would also conserve energy. Commonly, an end-product such as D will shut off an enzyme early in the pathway, such as E1. This is called **negative feedback**, or **feedback inhibition**.

Figure 15   Feedback Inhibition

There are examples of positive feedback ("feedback *stimulation*"), but negative feedback is by far the most common example of feedback regulation. On the other hand, *feedforward stimulation* is common. This involves the stimulation of an enzyme by its substrate or by a molecule used in the synthesis of the substrate. For example, in Figure 15, A might stimulate E3. This makes sense because when lots of A is around, we want the pathway for utilization of A to be active.

Allosteric regulation can be quite complex. It is possible for more than one small molecule to be capable of binding to an allosteric site. For example, imagine a reaction pathway from A through Z, in which each step (A → B, B → C, etc.) is catalyzed by an enzyme. Let's say that an allosteric enzyme called E15 catalyzes the reaction O → P. It would be possible for A to allosterically activate E15 (feedforward stimulation) and for Z to allosterically inhibit E15 (feedback inhibition). This may sound complex, but it's quite logical. What it means is that when lots of A is around, E15 will be stimulated to use the molecules made from A (B, C, D, etc.) to make P, which could then be used to make Q, R, S, etc., all the way up to Z. On the other hand, if a lot of excess Z built up, it would inhibit E15, thereby conserving the supply of A, B, C, etc. and preventing more build-up of Z, Y, X, etc. Therefore, in addition to acting as switches, enzymes act as *valves*, because they regulate the flow of substrates into products.

4.7 ENZYME KINETICS

Enzyme kinetics is the study of the rate of formation of products from substrates in the presence of an enzyme. The **reaction rate** (*V*, for velocity) is the amount of product formed per unit time, in moles per second (mol/s). It depends on the concentration of substrate, [S], and enzyme.[34] If there is only a little substrate, then the rate *V* is directly proportional to the amount of substrate added: double the amount of substrate and the reaction rate doubles, triple the substrate and the rate triples, and so forth. But eventually there is so much substrate that the active sites of the enzymes are occupied much of the time, and adding more substrate doesn't increase the reaction rate as much, that is, the slope of the *V* vs. [S] curve decreases. Finally, there is so much substrate that every active site is continuously occupied, and adding more substrate doesn't increase the reaction rate at all. At this point, the enzyme is said to be **saturated**. The reaction rate when the enzyme is saturated is denoted V_{max} (see Figure 16). This is a property of each enzyme at a particular concentration of enzyme. You can look it up in a book for the common ones. [If a small amount of enzyme in a solution is acting at V_{max} and the substrate concentration is doubled, what is the new reaction rate?[35]]

Another commonly used parameter on these enzyme kinetics graphs is the Michaelis constant K_m. K_m is the substrate concentration at which the reaction velocity is half its maximum. To find K_m on the enzyme kinetics graph, mark the V_{max} on the *y*-axis; then divide this distance in half to find $V_{max}/2$. K_m is found by drawing a horizontal line from $V_{max}/2$ to the curve and then a vertical line down to the *x*-axis. K_m is unique for each enzyme-substrate pair and gives information on the affinity of the enzyme for its substrate. If an enzyme-substrate pair has a low K_m, it means that not very much substrate is required to get the reaction rate to half the maximum rate; thus, the enzyme has a high affinity for this particular substrate.

---

[34] Usually the concentration of enzyme is kept fixed, and [S] is taken as the only independent variable (the one the rate depends on). This is applicable to biological systems, where substrate concentrations change much more than enzyme concentrations.

[35] If the enzyme is acting at V_{max}, it is saturated with substrate; adding more substrate will not increase the reaction rate; the rate is still V_{max}.

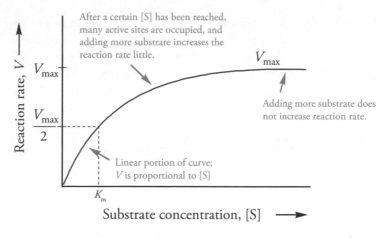

After a certain [S] has been reached, many active sites are occupied, and adding more substrate increases the reaction rate little.

V_{max}

Adding more substrate does not increase reaction rate.

Linear portion of curve: V is proportional to [S]

Figure 16 Saturation Kinetics

4.7

Cooperativity

Many multisubunit enzymes do not behave in the simple kinetic manner described above. In such enzymes, the binding of substrate to one subunit modulates the affinity of other subunits for substrate. Such enzymes are said to bind substrate cooperatively. There are two types of cooperativity: positive and negative. In positive cooperativity, the binding of a substrate to one subunit increases the affinity of the other subunits for substrate. The conformation of the enzyme prior to substrate binding, with low substrate affinity, is sometimes termed "tense," and the conformation of enzyme with increased affinity is termed "relaxed"[36] (Figure 17). Negative cooperativity (which is less important for the MCAT) is the opposite: the binding of a substrate to one subunit reduces the affinity of the other subunits for substrate. Cooperative enzymes must have more than one active site. They are usually multisubunit complexes, composed of more than one protein chain held together in a quaternary structure. They may also be a single-subunit enzyme with two or more active sites.

Figure 17 Positive Enzyme Cooperativity

---

[36] Imagine a group of people who can't get any dates. They are all depressed about it, and they keep each other depressed, which makes it even less likely that any will get a date. They are tense, "turned off," and inactive. Then one of the depressed group gets a date and gets so excited about it that all the other friends in the group get so enthusiastic that they get dates too. They are "turned on," relaxed, hip, groovy, and active.

A sigmoidal curve results from positive cooperative binding. In Figure 18 below, the flat part at the bottom left (Region 1) is explained by the notion that at low [S] the enzyme complex has a low affinity for substrate (is in the tense state), and adding more substrate increases the rate little. The steep part in the middle of the curve (Region 2) represents the range of substrate concentrations in which adding substrate greatly increases the reaction rate, because the enzyme complex is in the relaxed state. [The leveling off at the upper right part of the curve (Region 3) represents what?[37]]

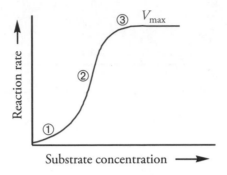

Figure 18 Sigmoidal Kinetics of Positive Cooperativity

Cooperativity does not apply just to catalytic enzymes. For example, hemoglobin (Hb) is a protein complex made of four polypeptide subunits, each of which contains a heme prosthetic group with a single O_2-binding site. (So one Hb has four hemes and four binding sites.) Hb is a carrier (of oxygen), not a catalyst of any reaction (not an enzyme). It exhibits positively cooperative O_2 binding. This is why the Hb-O_2 dissociation curve is sigmoidal. [What is the relationship between the two notions *allosteric* and *cooperative*?[38]]

---

[37] Saturation, just as in the case of a noncooperative enzyme.

[38] Cooperativity is a special kind of allosteric interaction. One active site acts like an allosteric regulatory site for the other active sites. Secondly, cooperative enzyme complexes are often allosterically regulated also. Hb is an excellent example. Not only does O_2 binding to one subunit increase the other subunits' affinities, but also several other molecules can bind to various sites to change the affinity of the complex. For example, CO_2 stabilizes tense Hb, causing each of the four binding sites to have a lower affinity for oxygen. As a result, in the presence of CO_2, Hb tends to give up whatever O_2 it has bound. The most important thing to remember, though, is that the binding in cooperativity takes place at the active site, while the binding in allosteric regulation takes place at "other sites."

4.8 INHIBITION OF ENZYME ACTIVITY

Enzyme inhibitors can reduce enzyme activity by a few different mechanisms, including **competitive inhibition, noncompetitive inhibition, uncompetitive inhibition,** and **mixed-type inhibition**. **Competitive inhibitors** are molecules that *compete* with substrate for binding at the active site. [You can predict that structurally, competitive inhibitors resemble what?[39]] The key thing to remember about competitive inhibitors is that their inhibition can be overcome by adding more substrate; if the substrate concentration is high enough, the substrate can *outcompete* the inhibitor. Hence, V_{max} is not affected. You can get to the same V_{max}, but it takes more substrate (see Figure 19). Therefore, the K_m of the reaction to which a competitive inhibitor has been added is increased compared to the K_m of the uninhibited reaction. [If an enzyme has a reaction rate of 1 μmole/min at a substrate concentration of 50 μM and a rate of 10 μmole/min at a substrate concentration of 100 μM, does this indicate the presence of a competitive inhibitor?[40]]

Figure 19 Competitive Inhibition

Noncompetitive inhibitors bind at an allosteric site, not at the active site. No matter how much substrate you add, the inhibitor will not be displaced from its site of action (see Figure 20). Hence, noncompetitive inhibition *does* diminish V_{max}. Remember that V_{max} is always calculated at the same enzyme concentration, since adding more enzyme will increase the measured V_{max}. Addition of a noncompetitive inhibitor changes the V_{max} and $V_{max}/2$ of the reaction, but typically does not alter K_m. This is because the substrate can still bind to the active site, but the inhibitor prevents the catalytic activity of the enzyme.

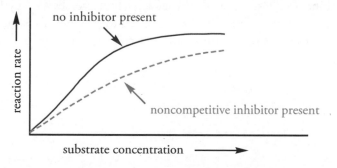

Figure 20 Noncompetitive Inhibition

---

[39] Structurally, competitive inhibitors must at least resemble the substrate; however, the most effective competitive inhibitors resemble the transition state that the active site normally stabilizes.

[40] No. The rate increase is greater than linear, indicating that the effect is caused by cooperativity.

- Carbon dioxide is an allosteric inhibitor of hemoglobin. It dissociates easily when Hb passes through the lungs, where the CO_2 can be exhaled. Carbon *mon*oxide, on the other hand, binds at the oxygen-binding site with an affinity 300 times greater than oxygen; it can be displaced by oxygen, but only when there is much more O_2 than CO in the environment. Which of the following is/are correct?[41]

  - I.   Carbon monoxide is an irreversible inhibitor.
  - II. CO_2 is a reversible inhibitor.
  - III. CO_2 is a noncompetitive inhibitor.

- In the figure below, the kinetics of an enzyme are plotted. In each case, an inhibitor may be present or absent. Which one of the following statements is true?[42]

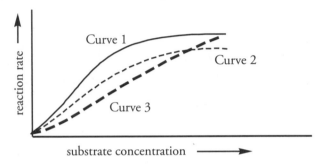

- A) Curve 3 represents noncompetitive inhibition of the enzyme.
- B) Curve 1 represents noncompetitive inhibition of the enzyme.
- C) The V_{max} values of Curve 2 and Curve 3 are the same.
- D) Curve 3 represents competitive inhibition of the enzyme, and the enzyme is uninhibited in Curve 1.

If an inhibitor is only able to bind to the enzyme-substrate complex (that is, it cannot bind before the substrate has bound), it is referred to as an **uncompetitive inhibitor**. Uncompetitive inhibitors, like noncompetitive inhibitors, bind to allosteric sites. This effectively decreases V_{max} by limiting the amount of available enzyme-substrate complex which can be converted to product. By sequestering enzyme bound to substrate, this increases the apparent affinity of the enzyme for the substrate as it cannot readily dissociate (decreasing K_m).

---

[41] Item I: False. The question states that CO can be displaced by oxygen. **Item II: True.** The question states that it dissociates easily. **Item III: True.** The question states it binds allosterically, which means "at another site" (not the active site).

[42] Since Curve 3 and Curve 1 have the same V_{max}, but Curve 3 has a reduced rate of product formation, it suggests that Curve 3 represents competitive inhibition of the enzyme in Curve 1 (choice **D** is correct). If Curve 3 represented noncompetitive inhibition, its V_{max} would be reduced compared to Curve 1 (choice A is wrong), and in no case would an inhibitor have a higher V_{max} than an uninhibited reaction (choice B is wrong). Lastly, it can be seen on the graph that Curve 2 has a reduced V_{max} compared to Curve 3 (choice C is wrong).

4.8

Figure 21   Uncompetitive Inhibition

Mixed-type inhibition occurs when an inhibitor can bind to either the unoccupied enzyme or the enzyme-substrate complex. If the enzyme has greater affinity for the inhibitor in its free form, the enzyme will have a lower affinity for the substrate similar to competitive inhibition (K_m increases). If the enzyme-substrate complex has greater affinity for the inhibitor, the enzyme will have an apparently greater affinity (K_m decreases) for the substrate similar to what we saw in uncompetitive inhibition. On the rare occasion when it displays equal affinity in both forms, it would actually be a noncompetitive inhibitor (many textbooks list noncompetitive inhibition as an example of mixed-type inhibition). In each of these situations, the inhibitor binds to an allosteric site and additional substrate cannot overcome inhibition (V_{max} decreases).

Inhibition Type	$V_{max, app}$	$K_{m, app}$
Competitive	no change	↑
Noncompetitive	↓	no change
Uncompetitive	↓	↓
Mixed-type	↓	varies

Table 3   Changes in the Apparent V_{max} and K_m in Response to Various Types of Inhibition

4.9   LINEWEAVER-BURK PLOT

The Lineweaver-Burk plot is a graphical representation of enzyme kinetics using the Lineweaver-Burk Equation:

$$\frac{1}{V} = \left(\frac{K_m}{V_{max}}\right)\left(\frac{1}{[S]}\right) + \frac{1}{V_{max}}$$

The equation may appear intimidating but can be interpreted as a simple linear equation of the form: $y = mx + b$. The graph is called a double reciprocal plot because the y-axis is the inverse of the reaction rate $\left(\frac{1}{V}\right)$ and the x-axis is the inverse of the substrate concentration $\left(\frac{1}{[S]}\right)$. The key aspects you need to know about the Lineweaver-Burk plot are the following:

1) The slope of the graph is $\frac{K_m}{V_{max}}$.

2) The y-intercept of the graph is $\frac{1}{V_{max}}$.

3) The x-intercept of the graph is $\frac{-1}{K_m}$.

Recall that increasing the substrate concentration ([S]) increases the reaction rate V up to a point. An increase in substrate concentration, however, is a *decrease* in the inverse of the substrate concentration $\left(\frac{1}{[S]}\right)$. Thus, an interesting aspect of the Lineweaver-Burk plot is that an increase in substrate concentration means a decrease in the value along the x-axis. Similarly, an increase in the reaction rate V is a *decrease* in the inverse of the reaction rate $\left(\frac{1}{V}\right)$. Thus, as the reaction rate increases, the value along the y-axis decreases.

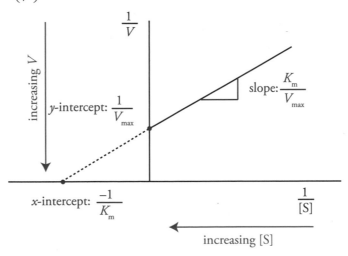

Figure 22   Lineweaver-Burk Plot

- How would the Lineweaver-Burk plot change when a noncompetitive inhibitor is added?[43]

---

[43] A noncompetitive inhibitor does not affect the K_m (so the x-intercept is unchanged) but does decrease the V_{max} (so the y-intercept increases and the slope increases).

Chapter 4 Summary

- Amino acids (AAs) consist of a tetrahedral α-carbon connected to an amino group, a carboxyl group, and a variable R-group, which determines the AA's properties.

- The isoelectric point of an AA is the pH at which the net charge on the molecule is zero; this structure is referred to as the zwitterion.

- Proteins consist of amino acids linked by peptide bonds, which are very stable. The primary structure of a protein consists of its amino acid sequence.

- The secondary structure of proteins (α-helices and β-sheets) is formed through hydrogen bonding interactions between atoms in the backbone of the molecule.

- The most stable tertiary protein structure generally places polar AAs on the exterior and nonpolar AAs on the interior of the protein. This minimizes interactions between nonpolar AAs and water, while optimizing interactions between side chains inside the protein.

- Proteins have a variety of functions in the body including (but not limited to) enzymes, structural roles, hormones, receptors, channels, antibodies, and transporters.

- Enzymes are biological catalysts that increase the rate of a reaction by lowering the activation energy.

- Unfavorable reactions in the cell are performed by coupling them to favorable reactions (such as ATP hydrolysis).

- Enzyme activity can be controlled via covalent modification, proteolytic cleavage, associations, or allosteric regulation.

- Competitive inhibitors bind at the active site of an enzyme, do not affect V_{max} but increase K_m.

- Noncompetitive inhibitors bind at an allosteric site of an enzyme, decrease V_{max} but do not change K_m.

- Uncompetitive inhibitors bind to the enzyme-substrate complex and reduce both K_m and V_{max}.

- Mixed-type inhibitors can bind to either the enzyme alone or the enzyme-substrate complex. They reduce V_{max} but have variable effects on K_m.

- The Lineweaver-Burk plot is a linear graph used to extrapolate the V_{max} and K_m of an enzyme. It is a visual aid that can be used to identify inhibitor type.

CHAPTER 4 FREESTANDING PRACTICE QUESTIONS

1. If a mutation changed an Arg residue in the protein interior to a Leu residue, what would be the likely effect on the ΔG of protein folding?

   A) ΔG would become more positive.
   B) ΔG would become more negative.
   C) ΔG would remain unchanged.
   D) The effect on ΔG cannot be determined without additional information.

2. Some inhibitors bind irreversibly to enzymes by covalent attachment. Would the kinetics seen under these conditions (V vs. [S] curve) be similar to those seen with a reversible noncompetitive inhibitor?

   A) Yes, because it would reduce the K_m of the reaction.
   B) Yes, because the net effect would be a loss of active enzyme available for the reaction.
   C) No, because if enough substrate binds to the active site, the reaction will reach V_{max}.
   D) No, because K_m will increase and V_{max} will stay the same, similar to competitive inhibition.

3. Some enzymes can modify their substrate, and by this means, regulate its activity. In many instances, these modifications are not permanent since other enzymes can reverse them. Which of the following category of enzymes will irreversibly modify their substrate?

   A) A kinase
   B) A protease
   C) A phosphatase
   D) An acetylase

4. Which of the following would have the LEAST effect on the ability of an enzyme to bind its substrate?

   A) Placing an enzyme that optimally functions at pH 7 in a pH 5 solution
   B) Increasing the temperature of the enzyme's surroundings
   C) Mutating the Glu and Asp residues in the active site to Lys and His
   D) Changing the substrate from a tripeptide to a disaccharide

5. For a given enzyme concentration at a low substrate concentration, how does reaction rate change as the substrate concentration increases?

   A) Logarithmically
   B) Linearly
   C) Exponentially
   D) Indirectly

6. Both hemoglobin and myoglobin are proteins that carry oxygen in the human body. Hemoglobin exhibits cooperativity and is found in red blood cells, whereas myoglobin is not cooperative and is found in muscle cells. Which of the following is likely true regarding these oxygen-carrying proteins?

   A) The O_2 saturation curve will be sigmoidal for myoglobin, but not hemoglobin.
   B) Hemoglobin has a lower binding affinity for oxygen than myoglobin.
   C) Hemoglobin is used to tightly bind oxygen in the body, while myoglobin is used to deliver oxygen to body cells.
   D) Hemoglobin most likely consists of multiple protein subunits, whereas myoglobin may or may not consist of multiple protein subunits.

7. Which of the following will be true of the Lineweaver-Burk plot of an enzyme in the presence of increasing concentrations of a competitive inhibitor?

   A) It will be a series of lines that intersect along the y-axis.
   B) It will be a series of lines that intersect along the x-axis.
   C) It will be a series of parallel lines.
   D) It will be a series of lines that will intersect, but neither on the y- or x-axis.

CHAPTER 4 PRACTICE PASSAGE

The Michaelis-Menten equation expresses the relationship between reaction velocity (V) and substrate concentration ([S]) for enzymatic reactions involving a single substrate.

$$V = V_{max}[S] / (K_m + [S])$$

Equation 1

Equation 1 yields a hyperbolic curve when V is plotted against [S] (Figure 1). Prior to the availability of computer programs that were able to perform non-linear regression, it was difficult to curve fit V vs. [S] data accurately to obtain values for K_m and V_{max}. To overcome this problem, multiple strategies were developed to represent the Michaelis-Menten equation in a linear form. One of the most commonly employed was the Lineweaver-Burk formulation (Equation 2), in which taking the reciprocal of Equation 1 yields a relationship that can be represented by a linear plot of $1/V$ vs. $1/[S]$ (Figure 1):

$$1/V = (K_m/V_{max}) \times 1/[S] + 1/V_{max}$$

Equation 2

Figure 1   Sample V vs. [S] plot with Lineweaver-Burk representation (inset)

Despite the advantages of this linear representation of enzymatic rate data, the Lineweaver-Burk plot introduces greater error when used to determine V_{max} and K_m. Thus, it is not recommended when highly accurate values of these kinetic parameters are desired. Instead, the continued utility of the Lineweaver-Burk plot lies in its ability to clearly differentiate modes of enzyme inhibition.

Many organisms employ enzymes related to complexes in the mitochondrial electron transport chain for oxidative transformation of environmental toxins. NADH oxidoreductase, isolated from *Methylococcus capsulatus*, is an example of such an enzyme that participates in the oxidative conversion of methane into methanol. In an experiment whose results are shown below in Figure 2, a researcher tested the ability of two different inhibitors to affect the activity of NADH oxidoreductase at two different concentrations. The results are displayed as Lineweaver-Burk plots.

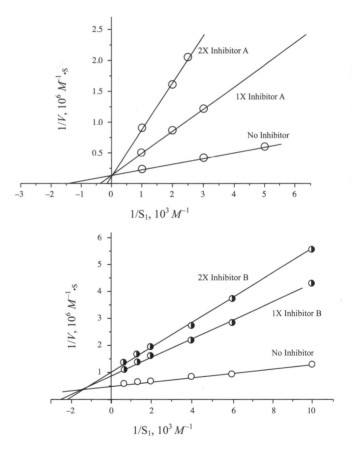

Figure 2   Inhibition of NADH oxidoreductase by two different inhibitors

Adapted from Saratovskikh, EA. *Kinetics and Mechanism of Inhibition of Oxidation Enzymes by Herbicides.* In Herbicides, Advances in Research. Edited by Price A and Kelton J. 2013

1. Which of the following is the best estimate for the V_{max} of the enzyme represented by Figure 1?

A) 0.02 μmol / min
B) 23 μmol / min
C) 44 μmol / min
D) 52 μmol / min

2. Which of the following represent possible sources of error when estimating K_m and V_{max} from a Lineweaver-Burk plot?

   I. The inability to obtain negative values of 1/[S] often requires extrapolation of the linear fit over a long stretch lacking data points in order to determine the x-intercept.
   II. Errors in the data obtained at low substrate concentration have a disproportionate impact on the determination of the best linear fit.
   III. Visual estimation of K_m and V_{max} is more challenging from a linear plot as compared to the hyperbolic plot of V vs. [S].

A) I only
B) II only
C) I and II only
D) I, II, and III

3. Which of the following is true concerning the slope of a Lineweaver-Burk plot in the presence of a competitive versus a noncompetitive inhibitor?

A) The slope changes in the presence of both a competitive and noncompetitive inhibitor.
B) The slope changes in the presence of a competitive inhibitor only.
C) The slope changes in the presence of a noncompetitive inhibitor only.
D) The slope does not change in the presence of either type of inhibitor.

4. Reductive detoxification of reactive oxygen intermediates is critical to the survival of aerobic organisms. Which of the following is most directly involved in this process in humans?

A) NADH produced by the pentose phosphate pathway
B) NADH produced by gluconeogenesis
C) NADPH produced by the pentose phosphate pathway
D) NADPH produced by gluconeogenesis

5. All of the following are true concerning Inhibitor A EXCEPT:

A) its effect on enzyme activity can be overcome by increasing the substrate concentration.
B) its effect on enzyme activity is equivalent to that of decreasing the concentration of the uninhibited enzyme.
C) it is unable to bind to the enzyme at the same time that substrate is bound.
D) its effect on enzyme activity is equivalent to that of decreasing the enzyme-substrate binding affinity.

6. Which of the following represents the Lineweaver-Burk plot of an enzyme alone (solid line) and in the presence of a noncompetitive inhibitor (dashed line)?

A)

B)

C)

D)

SOLUTIONS TO CHAPTER 4 FREESTANDING PRACTICE QUESTIONS

1. **D** Although the hydrophobic effect is a major driving force in protein folding, the favorability of protein folding is also determined by the favorability of amino acid interactions. Generally, the positively charged Arg residue would not be favored in the nonpolar protein interior, relative to the nonpolar Leu residue. The Arg residue, however, may be favorably interacting with an acidic residue in the protein interior. As such, without additional information about other interactions the Arg is involved in, the effect on ΔG cannot be reasonably predicted (choices A, B, and C are wrong, and choice D is correct).

2. **B** An irreversible inhibitor (regardless of where it binds) will permanently deactivate some enzyme, reducing effective enzyme concentration. If the enzyme concentration is effectively lowered, V_{max} will be reduced (choices C and D are wrong). This is similar to what is seen in noncompetitive inhibition, in which the inhibitor binds to an allosteric site and turns the enzyme off. Even if the noncompetitive inhibitor is reversible, because at any given time some enzyme is "off," the effective enzyme concentration is lowered and V_{max} is reduced. If K_m were affected, it would increase, not decrease; an increase in K_m indicates that the substrate-enzyme interaction has been compromised in some way (choice A is wrong).

3. **B** Proteases are enzymes that cleave their substrates at specific sites, permanently removing a part of the protein. This modification is practically irreversible—there are no enzymes that can reconnect proteins split by a protease. Choices A, C, and D are wrong because these categories of enzymes can reversibly modify their substrates. A kinase adds a phosphate to its substrate, but this modification can be reversed by a phosphatase that will remove the phosphate. An acetylase will add an acetyl group, while a deacetylase will remove it.

4. **B** Increasing the temperature of an enzyme's surroundings may or may not affect the likelihood of an enzyme binding its substrate. Increasing temperature will increase the kinetic energy of the substrate and make it more likely to enter the active site, unless the temperature is increased beyond the temperature of denaturation; since the question is not specific as to the magnitude of the temperature change, this is the choice that would likely have the LEAST effect (choice B is correct). Changing the pH of the solution to a non-optimal value will likely affect the charge of the protein side chains and enzyme function (choice A is wrong). Mutating acidic residues to basic residues will change the charge of the active site substantially and likely affect the substrate's ability to bind to the active site (choice C is wrong). Significantly altering the shape and size of the substrate will decrease its ability to effectively bind to the active site (choice D is wrong).

5. **B** At low substrate concentrations, the reaction rate increases linearly as the substrate concentration increases (see curve below). At or near saturation levels, the reaction rate begins to level off and does not change regardless of how much substrate it added. This is called the maximum velocity of reaction rate or V_{max}.

6. **D** In order to exhibit cooperativity, a protein must be composed of multiple protein subunits that are able to interact with one another (or, less likely, it should have multiple active sites within the same protein); thus, it is likely that hemoglobin is composed of multiple subunits. Since myoglobin does not exhibit cooperativity, it may either be composed of one subunit or multiple non-cooperative subunits (choice D is correct). Cooperative enzymes usually exhibit sigmoidal curves; hemoglobin would be expected to exhibit a sigmoidal curve, but not myoglobin (choice A is wrong). Cooperativity is a phenomenon involving changes in binding affinity when a substrate is bound; thus, binding affinity between a cooperative protein and a non-cooperative protein is not directly comparable (choice B is wrong). Note, however, that at the typical oxygen concentration found in tissues (e.g., muscle), myoglobin would have to have the higher affinity in order to be able to "steal" oxygen from hemoglobin and store it. Since hemoglobin is found in red blood cells, it must be the delivery protein, while myoglobin in muscle cells is the storage protein (choice C is wrong).

7. **A** In a Lineweaver-Burk plot, the y-intercept represents $1/V_{max}$, and the x-intercept represents $-1/K_m$. Because competitive inhibitors do not change the V_{max} and instead increase the K_m value, a Lineweaver-Burk plot with differing concentrations of competitive inhibitor will show intersecting lines that share a common y-intercept (choice A is correct). A common x-intercept would be indicative of an unchanged K_m value, as in the case of noncompetitive inhibition (choice B is wrong). A series of parallel lines is indicative of uncompetitive inhibition (choice C is wrong). A series of lines with any common intersection point not on the axes is indicative of mixed-type inhibition (choice D is wrong).

SOLUTIONS TO CHAPTER 4 PRACTICE PASSAGE

1. **D** This question highlights a main advantage of the Lineweaver-Burk plot. If Equation 2 is considered in $y = mx + b$ form, it is clear that the y-intercept (b) represents $1/V_{max}$. Looking at the hyperbolic curve that we are all used to, in which V_{max} is approached asymptotically, choices A and B are clearly wrong. In particular, choice A is too small a number, and it represents the y-intercept of the Lineweaver-Burk plot, which is $1/V_{max}$, not V_{max}. Choices C and D both seem in reasonable range when looking at the hyperbolic graph, but estimation is difficult, as it has not completely leveled off at the highest shown substrate concentration. In the linear plot, this ambiguity is resolved as we are looking for the y-axis intercept. In this case, it occurs at just less than 0.02, so V_{max} is just greater than 1/0.02 or 50 µmol/min.

2. **C** Item I is true: as it is impossible to have negative substrate concentrations, a Lineweaver-Burk plot will never have data points in negative x-axis (1/[S]) territory. As such, extrapolation of the line back to the x-axis will occur over a stretch of graph lacking data points (choice B can be eliminated). Item II is true: data obtained at low substrate concentration (and thus higher 1/[S]; in effect, the points at upper right of the graph), which are likely to have more measurement error, have a larger role in determining the slope of the linear fit (choice A can be eliminated). Item III is false: the passage suggests that the impetus for creating the Lineweaver-Burk formulation was the lack of computer programs that could accurately perform non-linear regression (fitting the hyperbola of a V vs. [S] graph). Clearly, drawing a straight line through points is easier (choice D can be eliminated, and choice C is correct).

3. **A** This question requires recognition of the meaning of the slope of a Lineweaver-Burk plot. Equation 2 is conveniently written in $y = mx + b$ format, in which the dependent variable (y) is $1/V$, the independent variable (x) is $1/[S]$, the y-intercept (b) is $1/V_{max}$, and the slope (m) is K_m/V_{max}. Competitive inhibition increases K_m, while non-competitive inhibition reduces V_{max}. As both K_m and V_{max} contribute to the slope, both modes of inhibition will engender a change in slope of the Lineweaver-Burk plot.

4. **C** NADPH is not generated by gluconeogenesis, and NADH is not generated by the pentose phosphate pathway (choices A and D can be eliminated). While our cells use NAD^+ as an electron acceptor in the oxidative metabolism of nutrients, they employ NADPH as the electron donor in reductive biosynthesis and in the process of detoxification of reactive oxygen species. Production of NADPH by the pentose phosphate pathway is one of the important functions of this pathway for the cell. The other is generating ribose for nucleotide biosynthesis.

5. **B** If you evaluate the linear plot in Figure 2 in the presence of Inhibitor A, you can see that the y-intercept ($1/V_{max}$) is not affected by the inhibitor, while the slope (K_m/V_{max}) increases. Thus, you conclude that the effect of this inhibitor is to increase K_m while leaving V_{max} unchanged. This is the signature of a competitive inhibitor, which competes with the substrate for binding to the active site (choice C is true and can be eliminated). Because they compete, increasing the concentration of the substrate will overcome the effect of the inhibitor on the enzyme (choice A is true and can be eliminated). As K_m is a measure of binding affinity of the enzyme for the substrate, the increase in K_m caused by this inhibitor is functionally equivalent to a decrease in affinity of the enzyme for its substrate (choice D is true and can be eliminated). However, since V_{max} depends on enzyme concentration, and since this inhibitor does not affect V_{max}, choice B is a false statement and the correct answer choice.

6. **A** A non-competitive inhibitor binds to an allosteric site on the enzyme, effectively turning the enzyme off, but it does not affect the ability of the enzyme to bind substrate. Thus, V_{max} will be decreased and K_m will remain the same. On the Lineweaver-Burk plot, a decrease in V_{max} is represented by an increase in the y-intercept (if V decreases, $1/V$ increases; choice B can be eliminated). K_m is represented by the x-intercept; since K_m is the same, there should be no change in the x-intercept (choices C and D can be eliminated, and choice A is correct).

COMPLEX II SUBUNIT SDHD IS CRITICAL FOR CELL GROWTH AND METABOLISM, WHICH CAN BE PARTIALLY RESTORED WITH A SYNTHETIC UBIQUINONE ANALOG

Aloka B. Bandara, Joshua C. Drake & David A. Brown
BMC Molecular and Cell Biology volume 22, Article number: 35 (2021)

BACKGROUND

Mitochondria generate the majority of adenosine triphosphate (ATP) through the electron transport chain (ETC). Succinate dehydrogenase (Complex II) uniquely serves as a component of both the Krebs cycle and the ETC. As a component of the Krebs Cycle, Complex II catalyzes oxidation of succinate to fumarate, whereas in the ETC, it is one of two entry points for electrons, acquiring electrons from succinate and donating them to ubiquinone (CoQ). Thus, impairments in Complex II function can have severe consequences for maintaining energetic homeostasis. Mutations in Complex II subunits have been found in patients with mitochondrial respiratory deficiency, as well as a number of cancers. Therefore, an in-depth understanding of Complex II in energetic homeostasis and its viability as a target for treatment is warranted.

Complex II carries four protein subunits, all of which are encoded by nuclear genes. Two subunits, SDHA and SDHB, are localized on the matrix side of the inner membrane, and carry the binding site for succinate, three FeS clusters, as well as a flavoprotein bound to an FAD cofactor. The two remaining subunits, SDHC and SDHD, are hydrophobic and anchor the complex to the inner-membrane. Subunits SDHC and SDHD form the CoQ binding site of Complex II and serve as terminal electron transfers from Complex II to CoQ. In particular, mutation of SDHD has been noted in patients with paragangliomas and pheochromocytomas. Therefore, given the particular role of SDHD in anchoring Complex II to the inner-membrane, passaging electrons to CoQ, and noted pathologies, modeling SDHD dysfunction could be a valuable tool for understanding the role of Complex II in metabolism and developing novel therapeutics. To date, however, suitable models for molecular examinations of any Complex II subunit do not exist.

We successfully used a CRISPR/cas9 approach to mutate the SDHD subunit of Complex II in HEK293 cells, and characterized its requirement for mitochondrial respiration, ATP synthesis, and cell growth in vitro. Furthermore, we demonstrate the efficacy of the mitochondrial therapeutic idebenone to improve mitochondrial dysfunction in cells with SDHD mutation. Our results demonstrate the necessity of SDHD for energetic homeostasis and suggests it as a viable target for therapies aimed to improve mitochondrial function.

RESULTS

Construction of mutant HEK293△*SDHD*

The single guide RNA (sgRNA) sequences were designed based on the 609 bp long *SDHD* nucleotide sequence of *Homo sapiens*. A 118-bp site of the forward strand of *SDHD* was predicted as the most reliable for mutation. The guide strand predicted was TCTGTTGCTTCGAACTCCAG (Fig. 1a). The constructed mutant HEK293△*SDHD* was validated by Western immunoblotting. The predicted molecular weight of SDHD is approximately 17 kDa. Nevertheless, the antibody used for mutant validation was anticipated to produce an additional band of about 29 kDa as well on the blot from parent cells. Our mutant HEK293△*SDHD* was found missing both 17 kDa and 29 kDa protein bands (Fig. 1b).

A. GTTCGTTGCAACAAATTGATGAGCAATGCTTTTTTATAATGCC
AACTTTGTACAAAAAAGTTGGCATGGCGGTTCTCTGGAGGCTG
AGTGCCGTTCCGGTGCCCTAGGAGGCCGAGC**TCTGTTGCTTC**
GAACTCCAGTGGTCAGACCTGCTCATATCTCAGCATTTCTTCA
GGACCGACCTATCCCAGAATGGTGTGGAGTGCAGCACATACAC
TTGTCACCGAGCCACCATTCTGGCTCCAAGGTGCATCTCTCC
ACTGGACTAGCGAGAGGGTTGTCAGTGTTTGCTCCTGGGTCT
GCTTCCGGCTGTTATTTGAATCCTTGCTCTGCGATGGACTAT
TCCCTGGCTGCAGCCCTCACTCTTCATGGTCATGGGGCCTTG
GACAAGTTGTTACTGACTATGTTCATGGGGATGCCTTGCAGAA
AGCTGCCAAGGCAGGGTTTTGGCACTTTCAGCTTTAACCTTT
GCTGGGCTTTGTATTTCAACTATCACGATGTGGACATCTGCA
AAGCTGTTGCCATGCTGTGGAAGCTCTGCCCAACTTTCTTGTA
CAAAGTTGGCATTATAAGAAAGCATTGCTTATCAATTTGTTGC
AACGAAC

B.

C.

Parent: AGCTCTGTTGCTTCGAACTC**CAGTGG**TCAGACCTGCTCATA

Bases C and A have been deleted | Base G has been inserted

Mutant: AGCTCTGTTGCTTCGAACTC**GGTGG**TCAGACCTGCTCATA

Figure 1 Construction of the SDHD mutant. The gene sequence of SDHD with CRISPR targeting sites is shown **a**. Expression of SDHD protein is shown **b**. The protein extracts reacted with rabbit polyclonal antibodies to SDHD and rabbit polyclonal antibodies to β-Actin are shown. The DNA level recombination events in the genome of the mutant are illustrated **c**. Expression of representative subunits from all five ETC complexes are shown **d-i**. The expression of NDUFB8 (complex **i**; **d** and **e**), SDHB (complex II; **d** and **f**), UQCRC2 (complex III; **d** and **g**), MTCO1 (complex IV; **d** and **h**) and ATP5A (complex V; **d** and **i**) were normalized to the expression of β-Actin

We then PCR amplified and sequenced the *SDHD* region encompassing the CRISPR targeting site (at 118-bp) of the mutant. The results indicated that an INDEL mutation has been generated at a site two bases upstream of the GTT PAM sequence. Two bases (a C and an A) have been deleted from this site and one base (a G) has been inserted at the deletion site (Fig. 1c). As a result, the whole amino acid sequence downstream of this INDEL site has been altered. Moreover, a stop codon has been inserted 180 bases downstream of the GTT PAM sequence.

Using the online CRISPR prediction site of the Integrated DNA Technologies, we identified the top three potential off-target sites. The DNA regions encompassing these sites were PCR amplified and sequenced and were identical to those of the parent cell line indicating absence of any off-target genetic alterations in the genome of the mutant.

We then investigated whether mutation in *SDHD* altered the expression of other subunits of the five ETC complexes. Expression of complex II subunit SDHB (Fig. 1d and f) decreased significantly in the mutant ($p < 0.0001$) suggesting that SDHD expression has direct impact on expression of other subunits of the complex II. Moreover, expression of complex I subunit NDUFB8 (Fig. 1d and e), complex IV subunit MT-CO1 (Fig. 1d and h), and complex V subunit ATP5A (Fig. 1d and i) decreased significantly in the mutant ($p = 0.0249$, 0.0034, and 0.0073, respectively) suggesting an association in protein expression between complexes II and other ETC complexes. The expression of complex III subunit UQCRC2 (Fig. 1d and g) was not different between the parent and the mutant suggesting that mutation did not impact expression of this subunit/complex.

Loss of SDHD increases apoptosis and necrosis
Compared to the parent HEK293, the mutant HEK293Δ*SDHD* produced significantly increased amount of ROS at 0h (immediately after addition of the substrate to the reaction; $p = 0.0128$; Fig. 2a). Nevertheless, the mutant produced significantly decreased ROS amounts at 24h ($p = 0.0035$) and 72h ($p < 0.0001$) after addition of the substrate. These observations suggest that disruption of *SDHD* results in subsequent decrease of ROS generation over time. At all the time points, the mutant displayed significantly increased apoptosis ($p < 0.0001$, < 0.0001, < 0.0001, and $= 0.0043$ respectively at 0, 2, 24, and 72h post-incubation; Fig. 2b). The mutant also showed significantly increased necrosis ($p < 0.0001$ for each time point; Fig. 2c).

Fig. 2 ROS production, apoptosis, and necrosis of cell lines. ROS generation measured using ROS-Glo H_2O_2 Assay of parent HEK293 and the mutant HEK293Δ*SDHD* is shown (**A**). The measurements are expressed as total luminescence per 15,000 cells measured at 0, 24, and 72 hours after addition of substrate to the reaction. Apoptosis (**B**) and necrosis (**C**) per 15,000 cells measured using RealTime-Glo Annexin V Apoptosis and Necrosis Assay at 0, 2, 24 and 72 hours of incubation are shown. The apoptosis measurements are expressed as total luminescence, whereas necrosis measurements expressed as total fluorescence. Error bars represent the SE of the mean

Loss of SDHD impairs growth
After 4 days of incubation in growth media, the number of cells recovered from the mutant HEK293Δ*SDHD* culture was ~73% less than the amount recovered from parent HEK293 culture ($p = 0.0002$; Fig. 3a). The doubling of mutant over 4 days was significantly slower compared to that of the parent during the same duration of growth ($p = 0.0008$; Fig. 3b), suggesting that SDHD is vital for cell growth.

A.

B.

Fig. 3 Growth of cell lines. The number of cells harvested from the parent HEK293 and the mutant HEK293Δ*SDHD* cells after four days of the culture (**A**) and doubling times of cells (**B**) are shown. Error bars represent the SE of the mean

A.

B.

C.

Loss of SDHD impairs mitochondrial respiration

Mutation in SDIID decreased oxygen consumption all along the ETC (Fig. 4a). Complex I respiration was significantly decreased in mutant cells compared to parent ($p = 0.0019$). Subsequent to rotenone treatment, oxygen consumption of both parent and mutant decreased, but the oxygen consumption of mutant cells was significantly less than that of parent cells ($p = 0.0101$). In response to treatment with succinate, Complex II-mediated oxygen consumption was significantly repressed in mutant cells compared to parent cells ($p = 0.0002$), further confirming the effect SDHD mutation. The mutant also had decreased OXPHOS capacity ($p = 0.0002$) and maximal respiration ($p = 0.0017$). Oxygen consumption of permeabilized cells was also assessed (Fig. 4b). In the mutant, basal respiration ($p < 0.0001$; Fig. 4c), reserve respiratory capacity ($p < 0.0001$; Fig. 4d), and maximal respiratory capacity ($p < 0.0001$; Fig. 4e) decreased significantly. These assays collectively indicate a severe impairment of cellular respiration due to SDHD disruption.

Loss of SDHD impairs glycolytic capacity and ATP synthesis of cell lines

Extracellular Acidification Rate (ECAR) of intact cells was determined (Fig. 5a). Both glycolysis ($p < 0.0001$; Fig. 5b) and glycolytic capacity ($p < 0.0001$; Fig. 5c) decreased significantly in mutant cells. The findings indicate an association between SDHD function and glycolysis. The mutant cells produced significantly less ATP than parent cells at two different cell densities ($p < 0.0001$ when 3500 or 10,000 cells/well were used; Fig. 5d). Impaired ATP synthesis was consistent with suppressed mitochondrial and glycolytic metabolism.

Fig. 4 Respiration, of cell lines. Oxygen consumption rates in response to treatment with glutamate-malate (G/M), rotenone, succinate, ADP, and FCCP (**A**) are shown. The mean oxygen consumption rates were compared between the parent HEK293 and the mutant HEK293Δ*SDHD*. The *p* values for the differences between the mean values were 0.0019, 0.0101, 0.0002, 0.0002 and 0.0017, respectively for Complex I respiration, rotenone treatment, Complex II respiration, OXPHOS capacity, and maximal respiration. Oxygen consumption rate (OCR) was measured of parent cells treated DMSO (Parent + DMSO), mutant cells treated DMSO (Mutant + DMSO), and mutant cells treated 1μM idebenone (Mutant + Ideb). OCR per 20,000 permeabilized cells (**B**), and the calculated basal respiration (**C**), reserve respiratory capacity (**D**) and maximal respiratory capacity (**E**) are shown. The mean OCR values were compared between the parent versus the mutant or DMSO treatment versus idebenone treatment. Error bars represent the SE of the mean.

D.

Fig. 5 Glycolysis and ATP synthesis of cell lines. ECAR measured using 20,000 live cells/well (**A**), and calculated glycolysis (**B**) and glycolytic capacity (**C**) are shown. The mean values were compared between the parent HEK293 and the mutant HEK293ΔSDHD. ATP synthesis of parent and mutant cells measured using Mitochondrial ToxGlo Assay (**D**) is shown. The measurements are expressed as total luminescence per 3500 or 10,000 cells. Error bars represent the SE of the mean

Improved respiration and growth of HEK293ΔSDHD mutant cells treated with mitochondrial therapeutic idebenone

Idebenone is a short-chain benzoquinone with greater hydrophilicity, which has shown promise as a therapeutic for mitochondrial dysfunction. We tested whether idebenone modified oxygen consumption of mutant HEK293ΔSDHD cells. Treatment of permeabilized mutant cells with 1 μM idebenone significantly increased basal respiration ($p < 0.0001$; Fig. 4c) and maximal respiratory capacity ($p < 0.0001$; Fig. 4e), but not reserved respiratory capacity ($p = 0.8847$; Fig. 4d). In O2k respirometry assay, in the presence of succinate, idebenone was incrementally added 10 min apart, with concentrations of 1 μM, following by three subsequent injections of 5 μM each (Fig. 6a). Compared to vehicle (DMSO), 1 μM idebenone elicited a non-statistically significant increase in oxygen consumption ($p = 0.1250$; Fig. 6a). Subsequent dose of 5 μM idebenone significantly increased oxygen consumption compared to vehicle in mutant cells ($p = 0.0119$), which peaked after the second dose of 5 μM idebenone ($p = 0.0508$; Fig. 6a). After the final injection of 5 μM idebenone, OXPHOS capacity was measured by adding ADP. Idebenone treated mutant cells had significantly improved OXPHOS capacity compared to the DMSO treated cells ($p = 0.0148$) (Fig. 6a). We next investigated whether long-term idebenone treatment would influence cell growth. Due to the slow growth of HEK293ΔSDHD cells (Fig. 6b), cells were grown for 10 days in growth media where either 1, 5, or 10 μM idebenone was added to

the media. After 10 days, 25.4% more cells were recovered from cells treated with 1 μM idebenone compared to the DMSO control ($p = 0.00959$; Fig. 6b). However, treatment with 5 μM idebenone did not improve growth of the mutant ($p = 0.9433$; Fig. 6b), whereas treatment with 10 μM idebenone caused cell death (not shown).

Fig. 6 Restoring the defects of the mutant with use of the mitochondrial therapeutic idebenone. The oxygen consumption rates of permeabilized cells treated with DMSO or idebenone are shown (**A**). The rates per million cells in response to injection of substrates, inhibitor, or drug are depicted. The mean oxygen consumption values were compared between the idebenone treatment and DMSO control. The p values for the differences between the mean values of DMSO control versus idebenone treatment were 0.8689, 0.7605, 0.9394, 0.1250, 0.0119, 0.0508, 0.0323, 0.0148, and 0.1084 respectively for G/M, rotenone, succinate, 1 μM idebenone, 1st dose of 5 μM idebenone, 2nd dose of 5 μM idebenone, 3rd dose of 5 μM idebenone, ADP, and FCCP. The number of cells recovered from the mutant cultures treated with 1 μM idebenone or DMSO are shown (**B**). Error bars represent the SE of the mean.

DISCUSSION

We successfully used a CRISPR/Cas9 approach to mutate *SDHD*, a Complex II subunit in the inner-membrane region, in HEK293 cells, generating the first such model to study the role of this essential Complex II subunit. The INDEL recombination events at the 118-bp site disrupted or altered the whole amino acid sequence downstream of the PAM site. And, mutagenesis procedure did not create any detectable off-target genetic alterations. In agreement with the observed alteration of the *SDHD* DNA sequence, amino acid level expression of the protein SDHD was totally disrupted in the mutant. Moreover, as a result of the *SDHD* mutation, expression of another complex II subunit (SDHB) decreased significantly suggesting interdependency in expression among different subunits of this complex. Quite interestingly, the expression of a complex I subunit (NDUFB8), a complex IV subunit (MT-CO1), and a complex V subunit (ATP5A) also decreased significantly in the mutant suggesting an association in protein expression between complex II and other complexes. Nevertheless, the SDHD mutation did not alter expression of the complex III subunit UQCRC2 suggesting independency of this complex from complex II in terms of protein expression.

Mutation in *SDHD* disrupted respiration all along the ETC, suppressed glycolysis and overall ATP synthesis, as well as limited cellular growth. Importantly, acute treatment with the synthetic ubiquinone analog idebenone was sufficient to improve Complex II-mediated mitochondrial respiration, OXPHOS capacity, and cell proliferation.

Predictably, mutation of SDHD inhibited Complex II-mediated respiration. Interestingly, however, mutation in SDHD significantly reduced Complex I-mediated respiration as well. Since Complex II drives Krebs cycle in a clock-wise direction by converting succinate to fumarate, we hypothesize that mutation of SDHD slowed and/or disrupted Krebs cycle production of NADH, the substrate for Complex I. Mutation in SDHD also impaired OXPHOS capacity, maximal respiration, and ATP synthesis. Taken together, impairment in the SDHD subunit of Complex II is sufficient to impair overall ETC energy production.

Glycolysis, as determined by ECAR, was significantly reduced in HEK293Δ*SDHD* compared to parent cells. Reduced glycolysis may reflect a lower demand for pyruvate due to disrupted Krebs cycle as a result of mutation in SDHD, representing a potential negative feedback on glycolysis. Also, inhibition of mitochondrial respiration with oligomycin did not elicit a change in glycolysis in mutant cells, further reflecting impaired

mitochondrial respiration. In addition to the suppressed metabolism, we also noted significantly slower growth in mutant cells compared to parent cells in culture media, which is likely reflective of the metabolic impairment in mutant cells.

Mutation of SDHD increased apoptosis and necrosis. The impaired glycolysis and mitochondrial respiration may have weakened the cell and cell membrane of the mutant making the cells more apoptotic and susceptible to necrosis. Quite interestingly, the long-term ROS generation declined as a result of SDHD mutation. In general, electrons that do not follow the normal order of the ETC pathway and instead leaked out are eventually transferred directly to O_2 to generate ROS. In our SDHD mutant, it is possible that impairment of clock-wise direction of Krebs cycle may have decreased the synthesis of NADH and $FADH_2$, the two electron donors to the ETC. Thus, limited donation of electrons may have led decreased electron transport through the ETC as well as decreased electron leakage out of the ETC giving rise to decreased ROS generation.

Finally, we explored whether SDHD mutation could be bypassed to improve some of the phenotypes observed. Idebenone, is a short-chain benzoquinone that is more hydrophilic than ubiquinone, and has potential as a therapeutic for conditions associated with oxidative stress and mitochondrial dysfunction. Treatment with varying concentrations of idebenone improved Complex II-mediated oxygen consumption and OXPHOS capacity, suggesting that the ubiquinone analog idebenone is able to substitute for Complex II as an electron donor to improve ETC function. Interestingly, long-term treatment with 1 µM of idebenone increased cell proliferation in HEK293Δ*SDHD* cells whereas 5 µM did not. Idebenone is known to have cell-type specific effects on cell proliferation. While an increase in cell proliferation in our mutant HEK293Δ*SDHD* cells with idebenone is likely a result of improved substrate utilization, cell type should be taken into consideration for mitochondrial targeted therapies as to how other process may be influenced.

CONCLUSIONS

We generated a novel mutant of the Complex II subunit SDHD via CRISPR/Cas9 that resulted in severe augmentation to mitochondrial respiration and cell metabolism as well as suppressed growth. This novel tool could be valuable for testing potential mitochondrial-focused therapeutics as well as elucidating other mechanisms regulated by Complex II function.

METHODS

Cell lines and culture conditions

Human embryonic kidney cell line 293 (HEK293) were maintained in Dulbecco's Modified Eagle's medium (DMEM) supplemented with 10% (by volume) fetal bovine serum and 1% penicillin-streptomycin. Cells were sustained in a humidified incubator at 37°C and 5% CO_2. *Escherichia coli* were used for constructing the mutagenesis plasmid. Bacteria carrying the plasmids were maintained in Luria Bertani agar or broth, and sustained in a humidified incubator at 37°C.

Construction and validation of *SDHD* mutant

Disruption of SDHD synthesis was validated by Western Immuno-blotting using rabbit polyclonal antibody SDHD (1:1000 in blocking buffer) and rabbit polyclonal antibodies to β-Actin (1:10,000). A clone missing the protein bands representing SDHD was chosen for further work and designated as HEK293Δ*SDHD* (Fig. 1).

The DNA regions encompassing the top three off-targets were PCR amplified and sequenced.

Expression of protein subunits representative to each of the five ETC complexes was examined by Western immunoblotting.

Cell growth and metabolism

Aliquots of 100,000 cells of the parent HEK293 and the mutant HEK293Δ*SDHD* were introduced into 75 cm² flasks each carrying 25 ml growth media. After 4 days of incubation, cell numbers were quantified in triplicates.

Restoring the impaired growth and respiration of the mutant

Effectiveness of the potential mitochondrial therapeutic idebenone in restoring the growth defects of the mutant HEK293Δ*SDHD* was evaluated. In this procedure, mutant cells were cultured on 6-well plates at 2000 cells/well in DMEM medium supplemented 1, 5, or 10 µM of idebenone. Fresh media containing the drug was added on days 3, 6 and 9, and the cell counts in wells of triplicates was determined following 10 days incubation. Efficacy of idebenone in improving respiration of permeabilized mutant cells was measured by O2k respirometry.

Statistical analyses

Student's t-tests were performed. Mean differences between groups were considered statistically significant at $p < 0.05$.

Abbreviations

ETC: Electron transport chain
SDHD: Succinate dehydrogenase subunit D
OXPHOS: Oxidative phosphorylation
ATP: Adenosine triphosphate
CRISPR/Cas9:   Clustered regularly interspaced short palindromic repeats/CRISPR-associated protein 9
DMSO: dimethyl sulfoxide
ROS: Reactive oxygen species
OCR: Oxygen consumption rate

JOURNAL ARTICLE EXERCISE 1

The science sections on the MCAT include a significant number of passages with experiments. Questions for these passages often ask you to analyze data, read charts and graphs, and come to certain conclusions based on the information they give you. If you don't know how to extract information efficiently and analyze data effectively, you will be at a distinct disadvantage.

There are three "Journal Article Exercises" in this book. In this first exercise, we'll show you the type of information you should be able to extract from the article and the sorts of things to pay attention to in the data. In the subsequent exercise, you'll do more of that on your own, and in the final exercise we'll show you how that article might get turned into an MCAT-style passage.

When analyzing an experiment, you should be able to:

- identify the control group(s).
- extract information from graphs and data tables.
- determine how the experimental group(s) change relative to the control.
- determine if the results are statistically significant.
- come to a reasonable conclusion about WHY the results were observed.
- consider potential weaknesses in the study.
- determine how to increase the power of the study.
- decide what the next most logical experiment or study should be.

The goal of these exercises is NOT to learn content from the articles, just to get more comfortable reading and extracting information from them.

For the (abridged) article on the pages 99–106, try to summarize the purpose of the experiment and the methods in four to five sentences. Consider the following mnemonic: Oh ouR Car Won't Start (ORCWS).

- **O = Organism and Organization**: is the research being conducted on humans or on animals or on bacteria, or something else? What is being done to these organisms? Are there any unique qualities to these organisms? Are there multiple groups? Is the study conducted over a long period of time with multiple data points, or is it a short-term study? Does it have a large or small n?
- **R = Results**: where and how are the results presented? Is it a graph? A data table? Figures and images? What is/are the independent variable(s)? What is/are the dependent variable(s)? Do the results show correlation or cause and effect, or both? Describe.
- **C = Control and Comparison**: is there a control group? How does it differ from the experimental group? Is it given a placebo or nothing at all? Is it held under different conditions? If there are multiple experimental groups, how do they differ from one another? Is it a blinded study? If so, double-blind or single-blind?
- **W = Weirdness**: does anything or do any of the results stand out as unexpected?
- **S = Statistics**: was any sort of statistical analysis done? How is it presented? Are there error bars on a graph? Standard errors around a mean? Are there p-values? Is there an asterisk indicating statistical significance? Is there any data that is not statistically significant?

Try interpreting the data on your own before reading the results/discussion section. When you do read the discussion, consider:

- What are the conclusions of the study?
- How are the conclusions supported by the data?
- What potential weaknesses or flaws do you see in the experimental design? Are these addressed in the discussion section?
- How might this study be potentially biased?
- How might this study be improved?
- What would be the next most logical experiment?

SOLUTIONS TO JOURNAL ARTICLE EXERCISE 1

Let's answer the above questions for the article on pages 99–106.

1. **O = Organism and Organization:**
   - Is the research being conducted on humans or on animals or on bacteria, or something else? *Human cell line – human embryonic kidney, HEK293*
   - What is being done to these organisms? *The gene for Complex II SDHD (succinate dehydrogenase complex subunit D) is knocked out and mitochondrial respiration is measured in comparison to parent cell line.*
   - Are there any unique qualities to these organisms? *The knockout cell line was created via CRISPR-Cas9.*
   - Are there multiple groups? *Two: HEK293 cells and HEK293ΔSDHD cells*
   - Is the study conducted over a long period of time with multiple data points, or is it a short-term study? *Short-term study (72 hours)*
   - Does it have a large or small n? *Large n: just over one million HEK293 cells, just under 0.5 million HEK293ΔSDHD cells*

2. **R = Results:**
   - Where and how are the results presented? Is it a graph? A data table? Figures and images? *Graphs, images of sequences, and images of gels*
   - What is/are the independent variable(s)? *Time, presence/absence of SDHD*
   - What is/are the dependent variable(s)? *Cell growth, ROS levels, apoptosis, necrosis, oxygen consumption, glycolysis, ATP synthesis*
   - Do the results show correlation or cause and effect, or both? Describe. *Both. Correlation: Decreased cell numbers and increased doubling time for mutant HEK293ΔSDHD cells over parent HEK cells; Cause and effect: HEK293ΔSDHD cells demonstrated less ROS but more apoptosis and necrosis than HEK cells.*

3. **C = Control and Comparison:**
   - Is there a control group? *Yes*
   - How does it differ from the experimental group? Is it given a placebo or nothing at all? Is it held under different conditions? *HEK cells have SDHS intact*
   - If there are multiple experimental groups, how do they differ from one another? *Only one experimental group, HEK293ΔSDHD cells*
   - Is it a blinded study? If so, double blind or single blind? *Not a blinded study*

4. **W = Weirdness:**
   - Does anything or do any of the results stand out as unexpected? *It seemed unexpected that the 5 μM idebenone treatment was less effective than the 1μM.*

5. **S = Statistics:**
   - Was any sort of statistical analysis done? *Yes*
   - How is it presented? Are there error bars on a graph? Standard errors around a mean? Are there p-values? Is there an asterisk indicating statistical significance? *P-values, error bars, asterisks*
   - Is there any data that is not statistically significant? *Yes, difference in Complex III between HEK293 and HEK293ΔSDHD cells, difference between treatment with DMSO and 5 μM idebenone.*

6. **Interpreting the data:**
   - What are the conclusions of the study? *Mutations in Complex II can augment mitochondrial respiration and impair cell growth. As done in cell culture, this model could be used to test therapeutics for mitochondrial disorders and/or further explore the regulation of Complex II.*
   - How are the conclusions supported by the data? *The data shows significant differences in cell numbers over time between the mutated and control cultures. Additionally, measurements of cellular respiration show statistical differences between the mutated and control cell lines.*
   - What potential weaknesses or flaws do you see in the experimental design? Are these addressed in the discussion section? *Study represents an in vitro model that can isolate SDHD from Complex II and measure the isolated effect of its knockout but does not provide an in vivo comparison for this knockout.*
   - How might this study be potentially biased? *Sample bias: the study was conducted on one cell line and its knockout.*
   - How might this study be improved? *Repeated on a broader range of human cell lines*
   - What would be the next most logical experiment? *Determine a method to simulate knockout conditions in a small animal model.*

7. **Final Summary of Experiment and Results:**
   - *In this journal article the impact of Complex II's SDHD on mammalian cell growth and metabolism was explored using HEK parent cells and a knockout strain, HEK293ΔSDHD. Cell growth of both strains was measured with the doubling time of the knockout showing significant increase along with its rates of apoptosis and necrosis. Additionally, multiple measures of cellular respiration were taken including but not limited to oxygen consumption and ATP synthesis with the knockout again being found to be significantly impaired. Treatment with mitochondrial therapeutics negated this effect in the knockout and could be scaled for greater bioenergetic capacity.*

Chapter 5
Carbohydrates and Carbohydrate Metabolism

Carbohydrates can be broken down to CO_2 in a process called **oxidation**. Because the process releases large amounts of energy, carbohydrates generally serve as the principle energy source for cellular metabolism. Glucose can be stored as the polymer glycogen in animals and as the polymer starch in plants. Glucose in the form of the polymer cellulose is the building block of wood and cotton. Understanding the nomenclature, structure, and chemistry of carbohydrates is essential to understanding cellular metabolism. This chapter will also help you understand key facts such as why we can eat potatoes and cotton candy but not wood and cotton T-shirts, and why milk makes some adults flatulent.

Figure 3 The Polysaccharide Glycogen

- Which requires net energy input: polysaccharide synthesis or hydrolysis?[2]
- If the activation energy of polysaccharide hydrolysis were so low that no enzyme was required for the reaction to occur, would this make polysaccharides better for energy storage?[3]

5.3 INTRODUCTION TO CELLULAR RESPIRATION

When glucose is oxidized to release energy, very little ATP is generated directly. Instead, the oxidation of glucose is accompanied by the reduction of high-energy electron carriers, nicotinamide adenine dinucleotide (**NAD$^+$**) and flavin adenine dinucleotide (**FAD**). Each of these carriers accepts high-energy electrons during redox reactions (forming **NADH** and **FADH$_2$**) and are later oxidized when they deliver the electrons to the electron transport chain. This generates the proton gradient that is used to generate ATP. Both of these carriers can serve as enzymatic cofactors and fulfill diverse roles in biological processes. For instance, NAD$^+$ is required for activation of adenylate cyclase by cholera toxin, and FAD can associate with a protein to become a **flavoprotein**. Dozens of flavoproteins have been characterized and are commonly involved in redox reactions (e.g., amino acid metabolism).

Glucose is oxidized to produce CO_2 and ATP in a four-step process: glycolysis, the pyruvate dehydrogenase complex (PDC), the Krebs cycle, and electron transport/oxidative phosphorylation. The first stage is **glycolysis** ("glucose splitting"). Here, glucose is partially oxidized while it is split in half, into two identical **pyruvic acid** molecules. [How many carbon atoms does pyruvic acid have?[4]] Glycolysis produces a

---

[2] Because hydrolysis of polysaccharides is thermodynamically favored, energy input is required to drive the reaction toward polysaccharide synthesis.

[3] No, because then polysaccharides would hydrolyze spontaneously (they'd be unstable). The high activation energy of polysaccharide hydrolysis allows us to use enzymes as gatekeepers—when we need energy from glucose, we open the gate of glycogen hydrolysis.

[4] The text states that glucose is split in half in the formation of pyruvate. Since glucose has six carbons, pyruvate must have three.

small quantity of ATP and a small quantity of NADH. Glycolysis occurs in the cytoplasm and does not require oxygen.

In the second stage (the **pyruvate dehydrogenase complex**), the pyruvate produced in glycolysis is decarboxylated to form an acetyl group. The acetyl group is then attached to **coenzyme A**, a carrier that can transfer the acetyl group into the Krebs cycle. A small amount of NADH is produced.

In the third stage, the **Krebs cycle** (also known as the **tricarboxylic acid cycle (TCA cycle)** or the **citric acid cycle**), the acetyl group from the PDC is added to oxaloacetate to form citric acid. The citric acid is then decarboxylated and isomerized to regenerate the original oxaloacetate. A modest amount of ATP, a large amount of NADH, and a small amount of $FADH_2$ are produced. Note that although the PDC and the Krebs cycle occur only when oxygen is available to the cell, *neither uses oxygen directly*. Rather, oxygen is necessary for stage four, in which NADH and $FADH_2$ generated throughout cellular respiration are reconverted into NAD^+ and FAD. The PDC and the Krebs cycle occur in the innermost compartment of the mitochondria: the **matrix**.

In stage four of energy harvesting, **electron transport/oxidative phosphorylation**, the high-energy electrons carried by NADH and $FADH_2$ are oxidized by the **electron transport chain** in the inner mitochondrial membrane. The reduced electron carriers dump their electrons at the beginning of the chain, and oxygen is reduced to H_2O at the end. (The word *oxidative* in "oxidative phosphorylation" refers to the use of oxygen to oxidize the reduced electron carriers NADH and $FADH_2$.) The electron energy liberated by the transport chain is used to pump protons out of the innermost compartment of the mitochondrion. The protons are allowed to flow back into the mitochondrion, and the energy of this proton flow is used to produce the high-energy triphosphate group in ATP.

Glycolysis

Glycolysis is an extremely old pathway, having evolved several billion years ago. It is the universal first step in glucose metabolism, the extraction of energy from carbohydrates. All cells from *all domains* (a domain is the highest taxonomic category) possess the enzymes of this pathway. In glycolysis, a glucose molecule is oxidized and split into two pyruvate molecules, producing a net surplus of 2 ATP (from $ADP + P_i$) and producing 2 NADH (from $NAD^+ + H^+$):

$$\textbf{Glucose} + \textbf{2 ADP} + \textbf{2 P}_i + \textbf{2 NAD}^+ \rightarrow \textbf{2 Pyruvate} + \textbf{2 ATP} + \textbf{2 NADH} + \textbf{2 H}_2\textbf{O} + \textbf{2 H}^+$$

Of course, it's not quite that simple. Glycolysis involves several reactions, each of which is catalyzed by a different enzyme (see Figure 4). The general strategy is to first put phosphorylate glucose on both ends and then split it into two 3-carbon units that can go on to the PDC and Krebs cycle. In the first step of glycolysis, a phosphate is taken from ATP and used to phosphorylate glucose, producing glucose 6-phosphate (G6P). This is isomerized to fructose 6-phosphate (F6P), which is then phosphorylated on carbon #1 (with the phosphate again taken from ATP) to produce fructose-1,6-bisphosphate (F1,6bP). This is split into two 3-carbon units that are oxidized to pyruvate, producing 2 ATP and 1 NADH per pyruvate, or 4 ATP and 2 NADH per glucose (since we get two 3-carbon units from each glucose). Don't forget that *each* glucose gives rise to *two* 3-carbon units that pass through the second part of glycolysis and into the Krebs cycle.

- An extract of yeast contains all of the enzymes required for glycolysis, ADP, P_i, Mg^{2+}, NAD^+, and glucose, but when these are all combined, none of the glucose is consumed. Provided that there are no enzyme inhibitors present, why doesn't the reaction proceed?[5]

Hexokinase catalyzes the first step in glycolysis, the phosphorylation of glucose to G6P. G6P feedback-inhibits hexokinase.

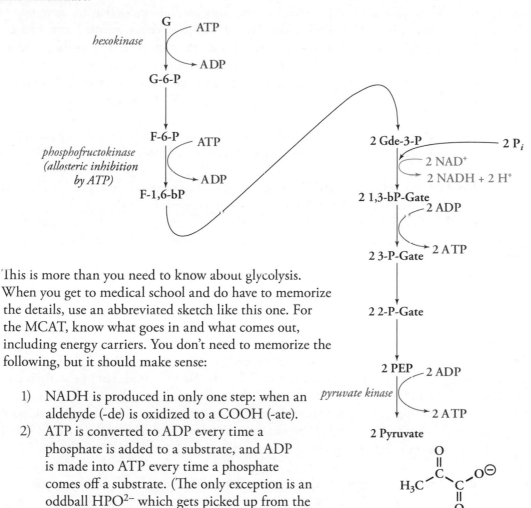

This is more than you need to know about glycolysis. When you get to medical school and do have to memorize the details, use an abbreviated sketch like this one. For the MCAT, know what goes in and what comes out, including energy carriers. You don't need to memorize the following, but it should make sense:

1) NADH is produced in only one step: when an aldehyde (-de) is oxidized to a COOH (-ate).
2) ATP is converted to ADP every time a phosphate is added to a substrate, and ADP is made into ATP every time a phosphate comes off a substrate. (The only exception is an oddball HPO^{2-} which gets picked up from the medium in Step 5.)

Figure 4   The 9 Reactions (Steps) of Glycolysis

---

[5] Although glycolysis results in a net ATP production, ATP is initially required to drive the reaction forward in the phosphorylation of glucose to glucose-6-phosphate and the phosphorylation of fructose-6-phosphate to fructose-1,6-bisphosphate. Without ATP to "prime the pump," there is no way to start the pathway. In case you're wondering about the Mg^{2+}, it's necessary for all reactions involving ATP.

5.3

Phosphofructokinase (PFK) catalyzes the third step: the transfer of a phosphate group from ATP to fructose-6-phosphate to form fructose-1,6-bisphosphate (F1,6bP). This is an important step because the reaction catalyzed by PFK is thermodynamically very favorable ($\Delta G \ll 0$), so it's practically irreversible. Also, G6P can be shunted to various pathways, but F1,6bP can react only in glycolysis. So once you light the PFK fire, you're committed to glycolysis. Therefore, PFK is the key biochemical valve controlling the flow of substrate to product in glycolysis, and the conversion of F6P to F1,6bP is known as a **committed step**. In the remainder of glycolysis, F1,6bP is split into two 3-carbon molecules that are converted to pyruvate, with the production of NADH and ATP. Very favorable steps in enzymatic pathways (those with a large negative ΔG) are practically irreversible (because the back-reaction is so unfavorable). These reactions are the ones that are usually subject to allosteric regulation. Another generalization about what steps get regulated is this: early steps in a long pathway tend to be regulated. This makes sense; if you're going from A to Z, it's more practical to regulate the A → B reaction than the W → X one.

For example, the enzyme PFK is a key regulatory point in glycolysis. PFK is allosterically regulated by ATP. [What effect would you think a high concentration of ATP would have on PFK activity?[6]]

Two molecules of NAD^+ are reduced in glycolysis per glucose catabolized, forming 2 NADH. As discussed above, NADH is an electron carrier, a molecule that is responsible for shuttling energy in the form of **reducing power** (i.e., reduction potential). Remember, these high-energy electron carriers are not used directly as an energy source, but are used later to generate ATP through electron transport and oxidative phosphorylation.

Fermentation

Under **aerobic** conditions (that is, in the presence of oxygen), the pyruvate produced in glycolysis enters the PDC and Krebs cycle to be oxidized completely to CO_2. The NADH produced in glycolysis and the PDC, as well as NADH and $FADH_2$ produced in the Krebs cycle, are all reoxidized in electron transport, where O_2 is the final electron acceptor. In **anaerobic** conditions (without oxygen), electron transport cannot function, and the limited supply of NAD^+ becomes entirely converted to NADH. [Would a limiting supply of NAD^+ stimulate or inhibit glycolysis?[7]]

Fermentation has evolved to regenerate NAD^+ in anaerobic conditions, thereby allowing glycolysis to continue in the absence of oxygen. Fermentation uses pyruvate as the acceptor of the high energy electrons from NADH (see Figure 5). Two examples of this process are (1) the reduction of pyruvate to ethanol (yeast do this in the making of beer, wine, etc.) and (2) the reduction of pyruvate to lactate in human muscle cells. Lactate is thought to contribute to the "burn" that athletes encounter during anaerobic exertion, such as sprinting, when the cardiovascular system fails to deliver enough oxygen to keep the electron transport chain running in muscle cells.

---

[6] When energy (ATP) is abundant, the cell should slow glycolysis. High concentrations of ATP inhibit PFK activity by binding to an allosteric regulatory site. It is interesting to note that since ATP is a reactant in the reaction catalyzed by PFK, you would expect a high concentration of ATP to increase the rate of the reaction (Le Châtelier's principle). However, the inhibitory allosteric effects of ATP on PFK outweigh this thermodynamic consideration. So lowering the concentration of ATP will increase the reaction rate, even though ATP is a reactant. Of course, if the ATP level went too low, the reaction could not proceed at all.

[7] If NAD^+ has all been converted to NADH, then the step in glycolysis that produces NADH (catalyzed by glyceraldehyde 3-phosphate dehydrogenase) cannot occur because it requires NAD^+ as a substrate. Thus, a lack of NAD^+ will *inhibit* glycolysis.

Figure 5 Anaerobic Pathways for Regeneration of NAD^+ from NADH

The NAD^+ produced by reducing pyruvate anaerobically is available for reuse in the glycolytic pathway, so more ATP can be produced. There is a limit to the use of anaerobic glycolysis as an energy source, however. The ethanol or lactate that is produced builds up, having no other use in the cell, and acts as a poison at high concentrations. Wine yeast die when the ethanol concentration reaches about 12 percent, and lactic acid is damaging at high concentrations in our tissues as well.

- What happens to the lactate in human muscle cells after a period of strenuous exercise?[8]

The Pyruvate Dehydrogenase Complex

The pyruvate produced in glycolysis in the cytoplasm is transported into the mitochondrial matrix, where it will be entirely oxidized to CO_2. Pyruvate does not enter the Krebs cycle directly, however. First it is oxidatively decarboxylated by the pyruvate dehydrogenase complex (PDC; Figure 6). **Oxidative decarboxylation** is a reaction repeated again in the Krebs cycle, in which a molecule is oxidized to release CO_2 and produce NADH. In oxidative decarboxylation, pyruvate is changed from a 3-carbon molecule to a __, while __ is given off and __ is produced.[9] The PDC changes pyruvate into an activated acetyl unit. An acetyl unit is [$(CH_3)(O=C–)$], and *activated* means the acetyl is not floating around freely but rather is attached to a carrier, namely **coenzyme A.** This coenzyme is basically a long handle with a sulfur at the end, abbreviated CoA-SH. It is used in many reaction systems to pass acetyl units around (e.g., fatty

---

[8] The lactate is exported from the muscle cell to the liver. When oxygen becomes available, the liver cell will convert the lactate back to pyruvate, while making NADH from NAD^+. Then the liver will utilize this excess NADH to make ATP in oxidative phosphorylation. This pyruvate can enter gluconeogenesis or the Krebs cycle in the liver, or it can be sent back to the muscle. (This cycle, whereby the liver deals with lactate from muscle, is known as the Cori Cycle.)

[9] Pyruvate is converted to a 2-carbon molecule, CO_2 is given off, and NADH is made from NAD^+. You can figure all of this out based on your knowledge of oxidative decarboxylation. Also, note the name of the enzyme, "dehydrogenase." To remove a hydrogen (*dehydrogenate*) is to oxidize. So the name of the enzyme also tells us that pyruvate is oxidized.

acid and cholesterol synthesis and degradation). When loaded with an acetyl unit, CoA-SH is abbreviated acetyl-CoA. The bond between sulfur and the acetyl group is high energy, making it easy for acetyl-CoA to transfer the acetyl fragment into the Krebs cycle for further oxidation. Regulation of the PDC is crucial. [AMP (adenosine monophosphate) is a low-energy molecule produced by the hydrolysis of ATP during metabolism. What effect would you predict a high level of AMP to have on the activity of pyruvate dehydrogenase?[10] The PDC is composed of three different enzymes. Why might a complex of three enzymes be more efficient than three independent enzymes?[11]]

Figure 6 Oxidation of Pyruvate by Pyruvate Dehydrogenase

Many enzymes require additional non-protein compounds for their biological activity. These molecules are called **cofactors**. Cofactors can be small (such as a zinc or magnesium ion) or they can be larger (such as a more complex organic molecule like NAD^+). If the cofactor is very tightly or covalently bound to the enzyme it is referred to as a **prosthetic group**. The PDC contains a thiamine pyrophosphate (TPP) prosthetic group at one of its active sites. The α-ketoglutarate dehydrogenase complex, which catalyzes the third step in the Krebs cycle, is very similar to the PDC; it has a TPP prosthetic group and catalyzes an oxidative decarboxylation. The **thiamine** in thiamine pyrophosphate is vitamin B_1. Vitamins often serve as cofactors or prosthetic groups.

- Beriberi is a disease caused by thiamine deficiency, which frequently results from a diet of white rice in underdeveloped nations. Which of the following would best describe the effect of thiamine deficiency on cellular metabolism in humans?[12]
  A) The rate of glycolysis would increase.
  B) Glycolysis would proceed anaerobically to maintain ATP production at normal levels.
  C) Glucose consumption would slow, and ATP production would increase.
  D) Acetyl-CoA would be provided by fatty acid metabolism, so the Krebs cycle would proceed uninhibited.

---

[10] A high ratio of AMP or ADP to ATP is described as low-energy charge. A low-energy charge will stimulate the PDC, increasing the rate of entry of pyruvate into the Krebs cycle.

[11] Simply because intermediates are passed directly from active site to active site, without having to diffuse.

[12] Thiamine deficiency would effectively shut down both the PDC and the Krebs cycle (choice D is wrong), since both of these processes require thiamine in their TPP prosthetic group. In the absence of PDC and Krebs, the amount of NADH and $FADH_2$ provided to the electron transport chain would be reduced, and ATP production would fall (choice C is wrong). In order to compensate and maintain ATP levels as close to normal as possible, the rate of glycolysis would increase (choice **A** is correct). Note that this would not happen anaerobically, as conditions are not anaerobic (choice B is wrong).

The Krebs Cycle

The **Krebs cycle** is a group of reactions which take the 2-carbon acetyl unit from acetyl-CoA, combine it with oxaloacetate, and release two CO_2 molecules. NADH and $FADH_2$ are generated in the process. The figure below shows an overview of the process; note that many of the names are not necessary to know and have intentionally been left out.

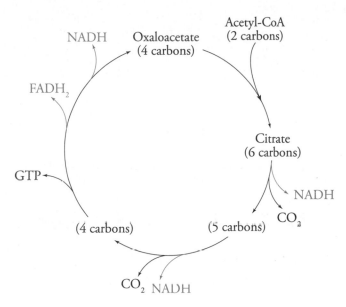

Figure 7   Overview of the Krebs Cycle

These reduced electron carriers (NADH and $FADH_2$) go on to generate ATP in electron transport and oxidative phosphorylation. Two other names for the Krebs cycle are the **tricarboxylic acid cycle** (**TCA cycle**) and the **citric acid cycle**. Citrate is the first intermediate produced in the cycle, as soon as the acetyl unit is supplied. Citrate possesses three carboxylic acid functional groups, hence the term "tricarboxylic acid." We will now break the multistep cycle down into three general stages. The reactions are shown for conceptual understanding only; there is no need to memorize structures or details. At most, you might choose to memorize the names.

Krebs Stage 1: The two carbons in the acetate fragment of acetyl-CoA are condensed with the 4-carbon compound **oxaloacetate** (OAA; the name is worth remembering), producing **citrate**; see Figure 8. As you will see, the OAA is derived from the previous round of the Krebs cycle; it is recycled each time. [How many chiral carbons are present in citrate?[13] If pyruvate is radiolabeled on its number one (most oxidized) carbon, where will the labeled carbon end up in the Krebs cycle?[14]]

Figure 8   The Entry of Acetyl-CoA into the Krebs Cycle

---

[13] None, since none of the six carbons has four unique substituents.

[14] It will not end up in the Krebs cycle. Pyruvate's most oxidized carbon is a carboxylic acid, which is removed as CO^2 by the PDC.

Krebs Stage 2: Citrate is further oxidized (twice!) to release CO_2 and to produce NADH from NAD^+ with each oxidative decarboxylation (Figure 9). The two carbons that leave as CO_2 during these reactions are not the same ones that entered the cycle as acetate. Thus, the two original acetyl carbons remain within the Krebs cycle. They will be lost as CO_2 in later cycles. [How many carbons from the CoA component of acetyl-CoA enter into the Krebs cycle?[15]]

Figure 9 Oxidation of Citric Acid to Succinate

Krebs Stage 3: OAA is regenerated so that the cycle can continue. In the process, reducing power is stored in 1 NADH and 1 $FADH_2$, and a high-energy phosphate bond is produced directly as GTP. Here GTP plays the role normally reserved for ATP. This GTP will eventually transfer its high-energy phosphate bond to ADP, converting it into ATP. $FADH_2$ is similar to NADH, but ultimately results in the production of less ATP.

Figure 10 Succinyl CoA to OAA

To review, the oxidation of glucose has so far created:

1) 2 ATP and 2 NADH per glucose molecule in glycolysis
2) Pyruvate Dehydrogenase: 2 NADH per glucose (one per pyruvate)
3) Krebs cycle: 6 NADH, 2 $FADH_2$, and 2 GTP per glucose

Thus, most of the energy of glucose is not extracted directly as ATP (or GTP) but in high-energy electron carriers. We will see how ATP is generated from NADH and $FADH_2$ in electron transport/oxidative phosphorylation.

---

[15] None. CoA assists in catalysis, which means that it is not consumed in the reaction, but regenerated as CoA-SH.

Compartmentalization of Glucose Catabolism in Eukaryotes: The Mitochondria

To understand oxidative phosphorylation, you must know the structure of the mitochondrion (Figure 11). The mitochondrion contains two membranes, an **outer membrane** and an **inner membrane**, each composed of a lipid bilayer. The outer membrane is smooth and contains large pores formed by **porin** proteins. The inner membrane is impermeable, even to very small items like H^+, and is densely folded into structures termed **cristae**. The cristae extend into the **matrix**, which is the innermost space of the mitochondrion. The space between the two membranes, the **intermembrane space**, is continuous with the cytoplasm due to the large pores in the outer membrane. The enzymes of the Krebs cycle and the pyruvate dehydrogenase complex are located in the matrix, and those of the electron transport chain and ATP synthase involved in oxidative phosphorylation are bound to the inner mitochondrial membrane.

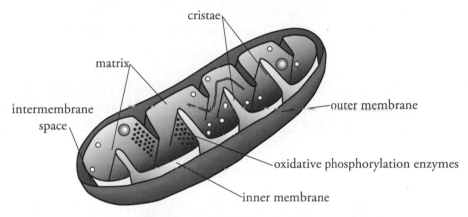

Figure 11 The Mitochondrion

The two goals of electron transport/oxidative phosphorylation are to:

1) reoxidize all the electron carriers reduced in glycolysis, PDC, and the Krebs cycle, and
2) store energy in the form of ATP in the process.

Where are all the reduced electron carriers located? Per each glucose catabolized, two NADH are created by glycolysis in the cytoplasm; the electrons from these NADH will have to be transported into the mitochondria before they can be passed along the electron transport chain. All the other NADHs and $FADH_2$s were produced inside the mitochondrial matrix, so they are in the right place to donate electrons to the electron transport chain.

The situation in prokaryotes is a bit different: all of the reduced electron carriers are located in the cytoplasm. In fact, everything is located in the cytoplasm, since there are *no membrane-bound organelles at all* in prokaryotes (no mitochondria, no nucleus, no lysosomes—everything just floats around in the cytoplasm). Since they have no mitochondria, can bacteria perform oxidative phosphorylation? *Yes, they can!* The way the process works is that a proton gradient must be created and then used to power ATP synthesis by the membrane-bound **ATP synthase**. So all that's required is a membrane impermeable to protons. Eukaryotes use the inner mitochondrial membrane; bacteria just use their cell membrane. The end result of this difference is that when eukaryotes perform aerobic respiration, they have to shuttle the electrons from cytosolic NADH into the mitochondrial matrix (at the cost of some energy), but bacteria do not. So, all things considered, prokaryotes get two more high-energy phosphate bonds from aerobic respiration than eukaryotes do (this will be discussed in more detail in just a bit). From this point forward, we will discuss the eukaryotic system. Remember that it's the same in prokaryotes except that they do it on the cell membrane instead of on the inner mitochondrial membrane.

Electron Transport and Oxidative Phosphorylation

Oxidative phosphorylation is the oxidation of the high-energy electron carriers NADH and $FADH_2$ coupled to the phosphorylation of ADP to produce ATP. The energy released through oxidation of NADH and $FADH_2$ by the electron transport chain is used to pump protons out of the mitochondrial matrix and into the intermembrane space. This proton gradient is the source of energy used to drive the phosphorylation of ADP to ATP. The **electron-transport chain** is a group of five electron carriers (Figure 12). Each member of the chain reduces the next member down the line. All five are named for their redox roles. Three of them are large protein complexes found embedded in the inner mitochondrial membrane. They are classified as **cytochromes** due to the presence of a heme group, a porphyrin ring containing a tightly bound iron atom. The other two members of the electron transport chain are small mobile electron carriers. The chain is organized so that the first large carrier receives electrons (reducing power) from NADH; the NADH is thus oxidized to NAD^+. Hence, the first large carrier in the e^- transport chain ("A" in the figure) is called **NADH dehydrogenase**. It passes its electrons to one of the small carriers in the transport chain, called **ubiquinone**, also known as **coenzyme Q**.[16] NADH dehydrogenase is also known as **coenzyme Q reductase**.

Cytoplasm

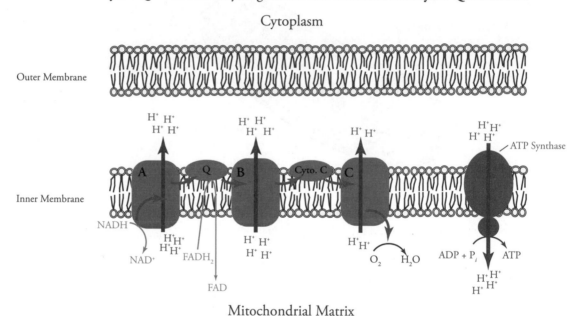

Figure 12 The Electron Transport Chain

Ubiquinone then passes its electrons to the second large membrane-bound complex in the chain ("B"), known as **cytochrome C reductase**. From this name, you can guess what the next carrier in the chain is called; it is **cytochrome C**, a small hydrophilic iron-containing protein bound loosely to the inner mitochondrial membrane. The last member of the electron transport chain ("C") is simply called **cytochrome C oxidase**. [Where does it pass its electrons to?[17]]

Each of the three large membrane-bound proteins in the electron transport chain pumps protons across the inner mitochondrial membrane every time electrons flow past. Protons are pumped out of the matrix, into the intermembrane space. The inner mitochondrial membrane is highly impermeable to protons. As a result, the electron transport chain creates a large proton gradient, with the pH being much __[18] (higher/lower) inside the matrix than in the rest of the cell.

---

[16] A quinone is a particular type of aromatic molecule, and the prefix "ubi" indicates that this molecule is ubiquitous, i.e., present in all cells.

[17] If it's the last member of the chain, it must pass its reducing power to O_2, reducing it to H_2O, an end product of electron transport. This is the only reason we breathe and the only reason we evolved with lungs, RBCs, etc.

[18] higher (remember, high pH = low $[H^+]$)

What does this have to do with ATP synthesis? Well, there is one more very important protein embedded in the inner mitochondrial membrane: **ATP synthase**. It is a large protein complex which contains a proton channel that spans the inner membrane. The passage of protons from the intermembrane space through the ATP synthase channel causes it to synthesize ATP from ADP + P_i. Thus, ATP production is dependent on a **proton gradient**. The overall process of electron transport and ATP production is said to be *coupled* by the proton gradient. Together, electron transport and ATP production are known as **oxidative phosphorylation**. Make sure you understand these questions:

- Dinitrophenol (DNP) is an uncoupler: It destroys the proton gradient by allowing protons to flow into the matrix. Which one of the following processes does it inhibit first?[19]
  - A) Pyruvate decarboxylation by the PDC
  - B) The TCA cycle
  - C) Electron transport
  - D) Muscular contraction

- Which one of the following processes has a positive ΔG under normal aerobic conditions in the cell?[20]
  - A) ATP hydrolysis
  - B) The pumping of protons to form a pH gradient
  - C) The oxidation of NADH by NADH dehydrogenase
  - D) The folding of a protein into its correct tertiary structure

- The reason cyanide is a poison is that it inactivates cytochrome C oxidase by binding to its active site with high affinity. When a person is exposed to cyanide[21]
  - A) the difference in pH inside and outside the matrix is already as large as it can become, so no more electrons can be pumped against the gradient.
  - B) anaerobic glycolysis depletes pyruvate, thereby slowing the Krebs cycle and the electron transport chain and slowing the rate of proton pumping.
  - C) the electron transport chain ceases to transport electrons and therefore ceases to pump protons.
  - D) NADH becomes fully oxidized by the Krebs cycle and therefore cannot reduce NADH dehydrogenase, so no protons are pumped.

---

[19] If the proton gradient is destroyed, the processes in A, B, and C will continue unabated, because NADH will be reoxidized to NAD^+ at a normal rate, or perhaps faster than normal. The problem will be that without a proton gradient no ATP will get made from all this glucose breakdown. The answer is choice **D** because this will be the first problem encountered from running out of ATP.

[20] Choices A, C, and D are all thermodynamically favorable processes that occur spontaneously without any external energy input. Thus, all of these processes have a negative ΔG. However, the large positive ΔG of the process in choice **B** makes undoing it favorable enough for it to power ATP synthesis. Creation of the proton gradient is dependent upon the very negative ΔG of electron transport.

[21] If the active site of cytochrome C oxidase is occupied with cyanide, then oxygen cannot bind there to be reduced to water; in other words, cytochrome C oxidase will be unable to get rid of its electrons and will remain reduced. Therefore, it will be unable to accept electrons from cytochrome C, which will be unable to accept electrons from cytochrome C reductase, which will be unable to accept electrons from coenzyme Q, and so on, all the way back up the electron transport chain. The end result will be a cessation of all electron transport chain activity (choice **C** is correct). Note that protons, not electrons, are pumped against their gradient (choice A is wrong), and this will stop completely, not just be slowed down (choice B is wrong). Also, NAD^+ is reduced to NADH in the Krebs cycle, not the other way around (choice D is wrong).

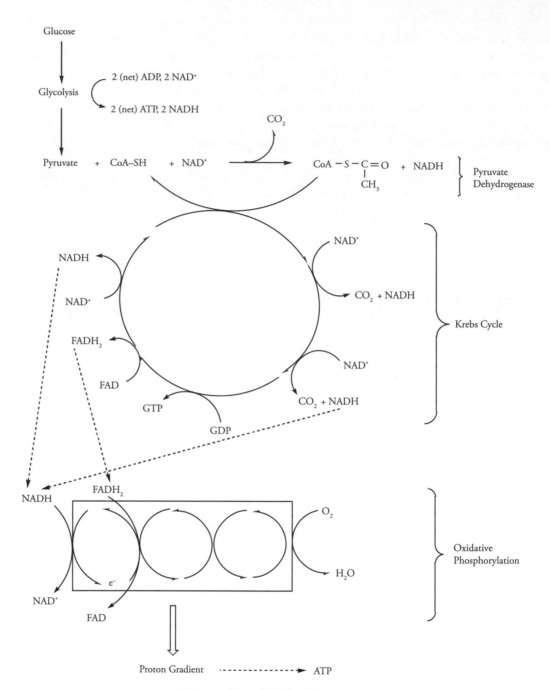

Figure 13   Cellular Respiration

Energetics of Glucose Catabolism

How is electron transport quantitatively connected to ATP synthesis? For every NADH that is oxidized to NAD$^+$, the three large electron transport proteins pump about 10 protons across the inner mitochondrial membrane, into the intermembrane space. The ATP synthase requires three protons to generate a molecule of ATP from ADP and P$_i$; however, an additional proton is required to bring P$_i$ into the matrix. This brings the "cost" of ATP synthesis up to four protons per molecule of ATP. Since NADH is responsible for the pumping of 10 protons, each molecule of NADH provides the energy to produce approximately 2.5 ATP molecules.

Even though NADH and $FADH_2$ have similar functions, their fates are a little different. $FADH_2$ gives its electrons to ubiquinone instead of to NADH dehydrogenase. By bypassing the first proton pump, $FADH_2$ is only responsible for the pumping of six protons across the inner membrane.

- How many ATP are made every time an $FADH_2$ is reoxidized to FAD?[22]

As mentioned earlier, the PDC, the Krebs cycle, and oxidative phosphorylation all occur in mitochondria in eukaryotes, while glycolysis occurs in the cytoplasm. The electrons from the NADH generated in glycolysis must be transported into the mitochondria before they can enter the electron transport chain. In most cells, they are transported by a pathway termed the **glycerol phosphate shuttle**. This shuttle delivers the electrons directly to ubiquinone (just like $FADH_2$ does), bypassing NADH dehydrogenase, and results in the production of only 1.5 molecules of ATP per cytosolic NADH, rather than the 2.5 normally formed from matrix NADH.[23] Bacteria, because they lack cellular organelles, do not need to transport cytosolic electrons across any membranes; hence the discrepancy in Table 1 in how much ATP is yielded from each NADH from glycolysis in eukaryotes compared to prokaryotes. All values in the following table are per glucose molecule catabolized.

Process	Molecules Formed/Used	ATP Equivalents
Glycolysis	–2 ATP 4 ATP 2 NADH	–2 ATP 4 ATP 3 ATP (eukaryotes) 5 ATP (prokaryotes)
Pyruvate Dehydrogenase Complex	2 NADH	5 ATP
Krebs Cycle	6 NADH 2 $FADH_2$ 2 GTP	15 ATP 3 ATP 2 ATP
Total		**30 ATP (eukaryotes)** **32 ATP (prokaryotes)**

Table 1 Theoretical ATP Yield from Cellular Respiration

Notes:

1) These numbers are an estimate of the theoretical maximum amount of ATP that can be produced from a single molecule of glucose. As the proton gradient is used to transport other molecules into or out of the matrix, the actual yield may differ depending on the number of protons (i.e., the gradient) available for ATP synthesis.

2) These numbers reflect the most recent understanding of ATP synthesis, and as such, may not appear in some textbooks that still cling to the previously established counts of 36 ATP per glucose in eukaryotes and 38 ATP per glucose in prokaryotes.

---

[22] Only 1.5 ATP are made as a result of the reoxidation of $FADH_2$. Six protons divided by four protons per ATP equals 1.5 ATP.

[23] Some high energy-requiring tissues (such as liver and cardiac muscle cells) utilize a different shuttle (the malate-aspartate shuttle) to bring the electrons to NADH hydrogenase, thus getting the full 2.5 ATP from those electrons. But this is the exception, and generally the MCAT does not test exceptions.

5.4 GLUCONEOGENESIS

Gluconeogenesis occurs when dietary sources of glucose are unavailable and when the liver has depleted its stores of glycogen and glucose (more on glycogen metabolism in a bit). This process occurs primarily in the liver (and to a lesser extent in the kidneys), and it involves converting non-carbohydrate precursor molecules (such as lactate, pyruvate, Krebs cycle intermediates, and the carbon skeletons of most amino acids) into intermediates of the above pathways where they ultimately become glucose. Gluconeogenesis is an 11-step pathway that uses many of the same enzymes as glycolysis. In simplified terms, it can be thought of as "glycolysis-in-reverse," in which those enzymes catalyzing the irreversible reactions (hexokinase, phosphofructokinase, and pyruvate kinase) have been replaced.

In Figure 14, starting from the bottom and working toward the top (i.e., starting with pyruvate), the first reaction of gluconeogenesis adds CO_2 to pyruvate, converting it to oxaloacetate. This step requires ATP hydrolysis and is run by the enzyme **pyruvate carboxylase**. In the very next step, oxaloacetate is decarboxylated and phosphorylated to form phosphoenolpyruvate (PEP); this step is run by **phosphoenolpyruvate carboxykinase (PEPCK)**. While this might seem odd (add CO_2 to then remove CO_2), oxidative decarboxylation is a favorable process, and it is often used to drive less favorable reactions. This same process is used in fatty acid synthesis as well (see Chapter 6).

The next several steps are run by the same enzymes as in glycolysis (PEP to fructose-1,6-bisphosphate). However, the phosphorylation of fructose-6-P to form fructose-1,6-bisP in glycolysis is essentially irreversible ($\Delta G \ll 0$), so it will require an enzyme other than PFK to reverse it. **Fructose-1,6-bisphosphatase** catalyzes the removal of a phosphate group from fru-1,6-bisP to form fru-6-P. This is then isomerized to glu-6-P and dephosphorylated by the final enzyme, **glucose-6-phosphatase** (as with fru-1,6-bisP, the reaction to form glucose-6-P in glycolysis is irreversible; therefore, its dephosphorylation must be run by an enzyme other than hexokinase). Furthermore, the dephosphorylation of glu-6-P is required in order for glucose to be released from liver cells into the bloodstream. Phosphorylated glucose is charged and cannot cross the cell membrane. This "newly-made" glucose can now travel to other cells in the body so that they can take it up and use it for energy.

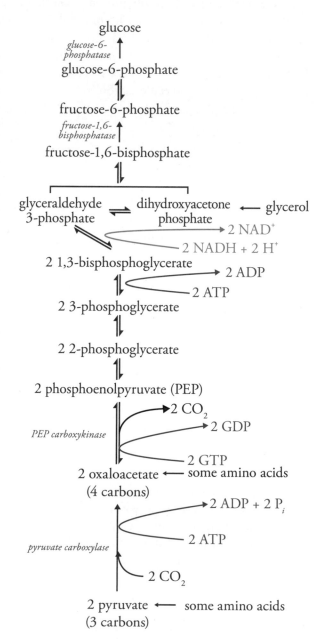

Figure 14 Gluconeogenesis

Altogether then, gluconeogenesis requires six high-energy phosphate bonds (four ATP and two GTP) and two reduced electron carriers (two NADH).

- As discussed previously, glycolysis is a thermodynamically favorable process with an overall $\Delta G < 0$. How is it possible for gluconeogenesis, which is seemingly the reverse process of glycolysis, to also be thermodynamically favorable?[24]

Note that while the majority of the intermediates discussed in cellular respiration can take part in gluconeogenesis, acetyl-CoA cannot. This helps explain why free fatty acids cannot be converted to glucose during periods of starvation, while the glycerol backbone of a triglyceride can.

5.5 REGULATION OF GLYCOLYSIS AND GLUCONEOGENESIS

Pathways that serve opposing roles (e.g., glycolysis and gluconeogenesis) must be tightly regulated to prevent the net loss of energy due to **futile cycling** (running both pathways at the same time). Therefore, **reciprocal control** in response to current cellular needs is critical. In reciprocal control, the same molecule regulates two enzymes in opposite ways.

As we already know, glycolysis and gluconeogenesis utilize many of the same enzymes. Attempts to regulate any one of these would fail to isolate a single pathway, so regulation must focus on those enzymes catalyzing irreversible reactions. Two such heavily regulated enzymes are **phosphofructokinase (PFK)** and **fructose-1,6-bisphosphatase (F-1,6-BPase)**. These enzymes serve opposing roles in glycolysis and gluconeogenesis, respectively. Both enzymes are allosterically regulated by glycolytic intermediates that activate one enzyme while inhibiting the other. For instance, in energy-starved states, elevated cellular AMP levels activate PFK while inhibiting F-1,6-BPase, resulting in enhanced glycolysis activity and a suppression of gluconeogenesis.

Another metabolic intermediate that exerts reciprocal control on these two enzymes is **fructose-2,6-bisphosphate (F-2,6-BP)**. Its intracellular concentration is set by a single large protein that functions as two separate enzymes: one that synthesizes F-2,6-BP and one that breaks it down. **Insulin** and **glucagon** help control the concentration of intracellular F-2,6-BP by regulating the activity of this large protein. Note that F-2,6-BP stimulates PFK (thus stimulating glycolysis) and inhibits fructose-1,6-bisphosphatase (thus inhibiting gluconeogenesis). To better illustrate how this works, let us consider an example. When blood glucose levels are high, insulin is released from the pancreas. Insulin stimulates the formation of F-2,6-BP, leading to the stimulation of PFK and activation of the glycolytic pathway. Simultaneously, the F-2,6-BP inhibits fructose-1,6-bisphosphatase, turning off gluconeogenesis so that these opposing pathways do not run at the same time. The reverse situation occurs when blood glucose levels are low; under these conditions, glucagon (also released from the pancreas) triggers the breakdown of F-2,6-BP. The drop in F-2,6-BP levels stops the stimulation of PFK, thus inhibiting glycolysis, and stops the inhibition of fructose-1,6-bisphosphatase, thus stimulating gluconeogenesis.

---

[24] There are three major steps in glycolysis with a $\Delta G < 0$ (the other steps have a ΔG close to 0). In gluconeogenesis, these same steps would have a $\Delta G > 0$. However, they are made thermodynamically favorable ($\Delta G < 0$) by coupling the reactions to the hydrolysis of the high energy phosphate bonds of GTP and ATP ($\Delta G \ll 0$).

- Following a high carb meal, the blood concentration of insulin _____ and glucagon _____.[25]

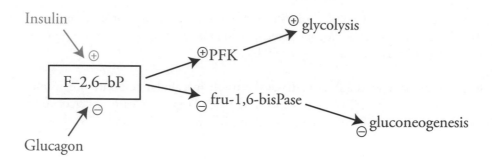

Figure 15   Hormonal Regulation of Glycolysis and Gluconeogenesis

Overview

In order to meet the varied metabolic demands of the cell, many additional forms of regulation occur beyond the limited examples outlined here. The following general principles, however, allow for reasonable predictions of the activity of a given pathway in response to cellular conditions:

1) In a pathway, those enzymes which catalyze irreversible (i.e., exergonic) reactions are frequently sites of regulation.
2) Increased concentrations of intermediates in a pathway generally serve to decrease the activity of that pathway (e.g., citrate decreases the activity of PFK in glycolysis).
3) Each pathway responds to the energy state of the cell. Cellular respiration is stimulated by energy deficits (e.g., high ADP:ATP or NAD^+:NADH ratios) and inhibited by energy surpluses (e.g., high ATP:ADP or NADH:NAD^+ ratios).

The table below outlines some of the regulatory steps described in this chapter.

Pathway	Enzyme	Positive Regulators	Negative Regulators
Glycolysis	Phosphofructokinase	Fructose-2,6-bisphosphate	ATP
		AMP	
Gluconeogenesis	Fructose-1,6-bisphosphatase	ATP	Fructose-2,6-bisphosphate
			AMP

Table 2   Summary of Metabolic Regulation

---

[25] Following a high-carb meal, the blood concentration of insulin increases and glucagon decreases. If you have a lot of carbs in your blood, you don't need to make any more!

5.6 GLYCOGEN METABOLISM

Glycogen is a polymer of glucose that is found in muscle and liver cells, and it is the main form of carbohydrate storage in animals. Glycogenesis, the formation of glycogen, starts with glucose-6-phosphate. The molecule is isomerized in a reversible reaction to glucose-1-phosphate by the enzyme phosphoglucomutase. Glu-1-P is activated with UTP to form UDP-glucose, which is added to the growing glycogen polymer by glycogen synthase.

Glycogenolysis starts with the phosphorylation and removal of one glucose unit at the end of the polymer, producing glucose-1-P. This is isomerized to glu-6-P, which can then reenter the glycolytic pathway. As in gluconeogenesis, in order to release the glucose into the bloodstream it must be dephosphorylated with glucose-6-phosphatase.

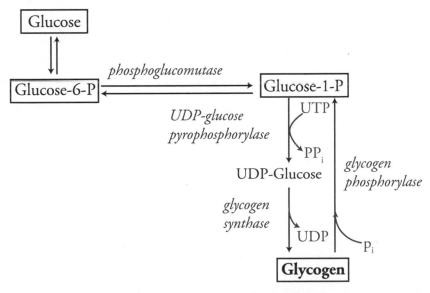

Figure 16   Glycogen Metabolism

Glycogenesis and glycogenolysis occur in both the liver and in skeletal muscle. Liver glycogen is broken down to maintain blood glucose levels during fasting states, while skeletal muscle glycogen is broken down to supply the skeletal muscle with glucose during exercise. Thus, skeletal muscle lacks glucose-6-phosphatase; the absence of this enzyme keeps the glucose phosphorylated and unable to leave the muscle cell.

Glycogenesis and glycogenolysis are opposing processes, controlled by the hormones that regulate blood sugar levels and energy. Insulin, released when blood glucose is high, stimulates glycogenesis. At first this seems paradoxical, as insulin was discussed above as a positive regulator of glycolysis (i.e., glucose breakdown), and it is not immediately apparent why breakdown and storage would be stimulated by the same hormone. However, it makes sense when you consider that it's unnecessary for all of the food just consumed to be immediately turned into energy, just as you don't necessarily need to spend your entire paycheck the moment you get it. You might spend some and put the rest in the bank. So insulin stimulates glycolysis (spending some of your paycheck) as well as glycogenesis (putting the rest in the bank).

Glycogenolysis occurs in response to glucagon, when blood sugar levels are low. It results in glucose being released from the liver into the blood where it can then be taken up by cells and enter glycolysis.

- Patients with Von Gierke's disease have a deficiency in the enzyme glucose-6-phosphatase. What would you expect these patients' blood glucagon and insulin levels to be?[26]

5.7 PENTOSE PHOSPHATE PATHWAY

The **pentose phosphate pathway** (PPP, also known as the hexose monophosphate shunt) diverts glucose-6-phosphate from glycolysis in order to form NADPH, ribose-5-phosphate, and glycolytic intermediates. This cytoplasmic pathway is composed of an irreversible oxidative phase followed by a non-oxidative phase consisting of a series of reversible reactions. NADPH and ribulose-5-P (from which ribose-5-P is derived) are made in the oxidative phase, ribose-5-P and the glycolytic intermediates are formed in the non-oxidative phase.

NADPH, although sharing much of its structure with NADH, has a different cellular role and serves as an important reducing agent in many anabolic processes (most notably, fatty acid synthesis). It also aids in the neutralization of reactive oxygen species. Ribose-5-P is used to synthesize nucleotides, while the other carbohydrate intermediates can be returned to glycolysis. Therefore, the "shunt" part of hexose monophosphate shunt...glucose can be shunted out of glycolysis to generate NADPH and ribose-5-P when necessary, and the glycolytic intermediates shunted back in.

- In order for NADPH to be an effect reducing agent, should the ratio of NADPH to NADP+ in the cell be high or low?[27]

---

[26] Without glucose-6-phosphatase, patients with von Gierke's disease are unable to produce free glucose from glycogen (and gluconeogenesis). As a result, these patients would have low blood-glucose levels, leading to chronically high levels of glucagon and low levels of insulin.

[27] A reducing agent is a substance that causes other molecules to be reduced (and is itself oxidized). As NADPH is the reduced form of NADP+, you would want a high NADPH to NADP+ ratio. This would favor the oxidation of NADPH in order for other molecules to be reduced.

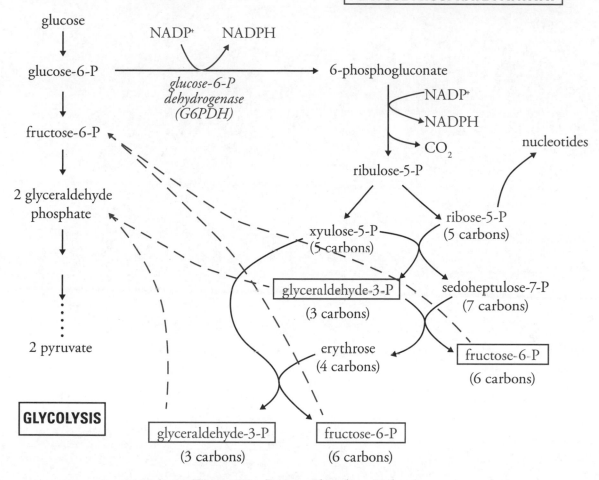

Figure 17 Pentose Phosphate Pathway

The first enzyme in the PPP, **glucose-6-phosphate dehydrogenase (G6PDH)**, is the primary point of regulation. Its product, NADPH, acts via negative feedback to inhibit G6PDH. The two successive oxidations in this part of the pathway (thus the name "oxidative phase") generate 2 NADPH. A deficiency of this enzyme (which is a common heritable disease) limits the ability of red blood cells to eliminate reactive oxygen species; this can lead to cell death and potential renal and hepatic complications.

Chapter 5 Summary

- Cellular respiration is the oxidation of carbohydrates, reduction of electron carriers, and generation of ATP.

- Glycolysis occurs in the cytoplasm and generates two pyruvate molecules: two ATP and two NADH per glucose.

- Under anaerobic conditions, the cell performs fermentation to regenerate NAD^+ so that glycolysis can continue.

- The pyruvate dehydrogenase complex (PDC) functions in the mitochondrial matrix, converts pyruvate into acetyl-CoA, and generates an NADH.

- The Krebs cycle in the mitochondrial matrix generates six NADH, two $FADH_2$, and two GTP per glucose.

- The electron transport chain in the inner mitochondrial membrane starts with the oxidation of the electron carriers NADH and $FADH_2$ and ends with the reduction of oxygen and the generation of a proton gradient across the inner mitochondrial membrane.

- ATP synthase in the inner mitochondrial membrane uses the proton gradient to generate ATP (2.5 ATP per NADH from the mitochondrial matrix, 1.5 ATP per NADH from the cytoplasm, and 1.5 ATP per $FADH_2$).

- Both eukaryotes and prokaryotes perform cellular respiration, but prokaryotes use their plasma membrane for the electron transport chain and generate two more ATP per glucose than eukaryotes.

- Gluconeogenesis generates "new" glucose from precursors such as pyruvate, oxaloacetate, amino acids, and glycerol.

- In reciprocal regulation, a single molecule controls two different enzymes in opposite ways. This helps prevent futile cycles (opposite pathways running at the same time).

- Glycogenesis stores glucose as a glycogen polymer. This occurs in the liver and the skeletal muscle.

- During times of starvation, glycogenolysis in the liver produces glucose that can be released into the blood. When the glycogen is depleted, gluconeogenesis can generate glucose from precursors such as pyruvate, lactate, and Krebs cycle intermediates.

- The pentose phosphate pathway generates ribose-5-phosphate (necessary for nucleotide synthesis) and NADPH (necessary as a reducing agent during anabolic pathways).

CHAPTER 5 FREESTANDING PRACTICE QUESTIONS

1. In eukaryotes, the ultimate yield of ATP from NADH is lower when the NADH is produced by:

A) glycolysis.
B) pyruvate dehydrogenase complex (PDC).
C) the Krebs cycle.
D) electron transport and oxidative phosphorylation.

2. Glycogen is a polysaccharide of glucose molecules with $\alpha1{\rightarrow}4$ connections and $\alpha1{\rightarrow}6$ branches. Amylose, a glucose-storing polysaccharide in plants, contains identical linkages, yet is hydrolyzed more slowly than glycogen. Which of the following explains this difference?

A) Glycogen adopts a tighter conformation than amylose does *in vivo*.
B) Plant digestive enzymes are specific to β linkages and therefore digest the α linkages in amylose at a decreased rate.
C) Glycogen contains $\alpha1{\rightarrow}6$ branches every 8–12 monomers, whereas amylose contains $\alpha1{\rightarrow}6$ branches every 12–20 monomers.
D) Amylose's $\alpha1{\rightarrow}6$ branches require more energy to hydrolyze than those present in glucose.

3. Which of the following changes would lead to a long-term increase in intracellular glucose levels in liver cells?

A) Decreased production of glycogen phosphorylase
B) Type 1 diabetes mellitus, caused by destruction of the beta cells of the pancreas
C) Expression of an overactive isoform of the pyruvate dehydrogenase complex (PDC)
D) Overexpression of pyruvate carboxylase

4. Salicylic acid (aspirin), if taken in excess, may act as an *uncoupling agent*. Uncoupling agents increase the permeability of the inner mitochondrial membrane, resulting in the dissipation of the proton gradient. Which of the following would most likely be true in the presence of an uncoupling agent?

A) Electron transport at the inner mitochondrial membrane would cease.
B) The energy from the proton-motive force would likely be dissipated as heat rather than in producing ATP from ADP.
C) H^+ ions would flow through the inner membrane into the intermembrane space.
D) There would be an increase in biosynthesis.

5. Which of the following is FALSE regarding the pentose phosphate pathway?

A) A decrease in the $NADPH{:}NADP^+$ ratio will activate the pentose phosphate pathway.
B) The pentose phosphate pathway would be upregulated during fatty acid synthesis.
C) The pentose phosphate pathway is most active during the M phase of the cell cycle.
D) A decrease in the pentose phosphate pathway activity may cause hemolytic anemia (premature destruction of red blood cells).

6. Glycogen metabolism is regulated by different hormones that activate reciprocal pathways. After several hours of fasting, a person eats a large meal. Which of the following statements is correct?

A) Elevated glucagon levels deactivate glycogen phosphorylase and activate glycogen synthase.
B) Elevated insulin levels deactivate glycogen phosphorylase and activate glycogen synthase.
C) Elevated glucagon levels activate glycogen phosphorylase and deactivate glycogen synthase.
D) Elevated insulin levels activate glycogen phosphorylase and deactivate glycogen synthase.

7. Which of the following is a product of the pentose phosphate pathway?

A) NADH
B) NADPH
C) Succinyl-CoA
D) Fructose-1,6-bisphosphate

CHAPTER 5 PRACTICE PASSAGE

Glycogen storage diseases (GSDs) result from the inappropriate synthesis or breakdown of glycogen. There are numerous types of GSDs caused by the production of dysfunctional or nonfunctional enzymes involved in glycogen metabolism. GSD V, commonly referred to as McArdle's disease, is caused by a deficiency in muscle glycogen phosphorylase, a key enzyme used in glycogenolysis. Patients with GSD V typically exhibit elevated levels of myoglobin in the urine and experience fatigue during the first 15 minutes of exercise followed by a sudden increase in the tolerance of exercise known as the "second wind" phenomenon.

Various tests are performed on patients with McArdle's disease to confirm the diagnosis. In addition to checking creatine kinase levels, patients will often undergo an ischemic (or non-ischemic) forearm exercise test. During an ischemic forearm exercise test, a blood pressure cuff is placed on the patient's upper arm and inflated to a pressure greater than systolic pressure, stopping blood flow to the lower arm. The patient then repeatedly clenches and unclenches their fist until they fatigue. Ammonia and lactate levels from the exercised arm are taken prior to exercise and at regular intervals after the forearm fatigues. For the non-ischemic forearm exercise test, the same procedure is used without the blood pressure cuff.

A patient complaining of low exercise tolerance and muscle cramps was also experiencing episodes of dark urine after exertion. A diagnosis of GSD V was suspected and diagnostic tests were performed. The person's creatine kinase levels were found to be four times the normal level. The results of an ischemic forearm test are presented in Figure 1.

Figure 1 Ischemic Forearm Exercise Test

Adapted from Park H, Shin H, Cho Y, Kim S, Choi Y. *The Significance of Clinical and Laboratory Features in the Diagnosis of Glycogen Storage Disease Type V: A Case Report.* JKMS: 2014; 7:1021-1024.

1. Which of the following best explains the changes in lactate levels after the first minute of the ischemic forearm test shown in Figure 1?

A) Depletion of NAD$^+$
B) Depletion of glycogen stores
C) Depletion of glucose
D) Depletion of ADP

2. Which of the following is/are expected be elevated in the muscle cells of a patient with GSD V?

   I. Glycogen
  II. Glucose
 III. Lactate

A) I only
B) III only
C) I and II only
D) I and III only

3. The purpose of preventing blood flow to the forearm during the ischemic exercise test is most likely to:

A) encourage anaerobic respiration.
B) decrease blood pressure in the forearm.
C) prevent the delivery of glycogen to the forearm.
D) decrease the level of lactate in the forearm.

4. Would the results of the ischemic forearm test in Figure 1 contribute to a diagnosis of GSD V for the patient?

A) No, increased glycogenolysis should result in increased lactate levels.
B) No, muscle fatigue should result in decreased ammonia levels.
C) Yes, decreased glycogenesis will lead to increased ammonia levels.
D) Yes, decreased glycogenolysis will lead to decreased lactate levels.

5. Given that the generation of creatine phosphate from ATP and creatine occurs spontaneously under standard conditions, which of the following is true regarding creatine phosphate metabolism in the human body?

A) Under resting conditions, the generation of creatine phosphate is favored.
B) During strenuous exercise, the generation of creatine phosphate is favored.
C) The generation of creatine phosphate is not favored in the human body.
D) In the presence of low concentrations of ATP, the generation of creatine phosphate is favored.

SOLUTIONS TO CHAPTER 5 FREESTANDING PRACTICE QUESTIONS

1. **A** In order for the NADH produced during glycolysis to be utilized by the electron transport chain (ETC) in ATP formation, the electrons must be shuttled into the mitochondria (remember, glycolysis occurs in the cytosol and the ETC along the inner mitochondrial membrane). When shuttled in, the electrons are typically used to reduce coenzyme Q and bypass NADH dehydrogenase. This results in the pumping of fewer protons out of the mitochondrial matrix, and thus, ultimately, in fewer ATP being formed. The NADH produced by the PDC or Krebs cycle is energetically equivalent because both occur in the mitochondrial matrix. Thus, this NADH is immediately accessible to the ETC (choices B and C are wrong). Finally, note that the ETC regenerates NAD$^+$ rather than producing NADH (choice D is wrong).

2. **C** Because glycogen contains more $\alpha 1\rightarrow 6$ branches, glycogen is a more branched polymer than amylose. The increase in the number of branches provides ends for hydrolysis, resulting in an elevated rate of digestion relative to amylose (choice C is correct). If glycogen were to adopt a tighter conformation, its glucose monomers would be more difficult to access, and it would likely be digested more slowly than amylose (choice A is wrong). If plant enzymes were specific to β linkages, they would be completely unable to digest α linkages, rather than show slowed digestion rates (choice B is wrong). Since both glycogen and amylose contain identical linkages, there is no expected energy difference of hydrolysis (choice D is wrong).

3. **D** Pyruvate carboxylase is responsible for the conversion of pyruvate to oxaloacetate in the first step of gluconeogenesis. Over-expression of pyruvate carboxylase would increase the rate of gluconeogenesis, causing increased intracellular glucose levels (choice D is correct). If glycogen phosphorylase production were decreased, glycogenolysis would decrease, leading to decreased glucose production (choice A is wrong). Destruction of the beta cells of the pancreas would lead to insulin deficiency, a hallmark of Type 1 diabetes mellitus. The absence of insulin would prevent the cellular uptake of glucose, leading to lower intracellular glucose levels (choice B is wrong). An overactive PDC would decrease pyruvate levels, driving glycolysis forward and causing decreased rates of gluconeogenesis. This would lower intracellular glucose (choice C is wrong).

4. **B** The proton gradient obtained by the electron transport chain (which pumps H$^+$ ions across the inner membrane into the intermembrane space) is necessary in order to create ATP at the ATP synthase. This enzyme allows the protons to move through its channel back into the matrix, and thus harnesses the energy created by the gradient to create ATP from ADP + P$_i$. If the inner membrane was made more permeable by uncoupling agents, then the H$^+$ ions would naturally move down their gradient, from the intermembrane space back to the mitochondrial matrix (choice C is wrong). This unharnessed energy would be dissipated as heat (known as non-exercise activity thermogenesis [NEAT]), and since the ions would not pass through the ATP synthase, less ATP would be created (choice B is correct). Although the utility of the electron transport chain would be compromised, the uncoupling agent would not inhibit electron transport itself (choice A is wrong); in fact this would lead to the rapid oxidation of Krebs cycle substrates and would promote the mobilization of carbohydrates and fats. Since the energy is lost as heat, biosynthesis is not promoted (choice D is wrong), and weight loss can be dramatic. Experimental uncoupling agents have been used in the past as effective diet pills; however, their use is very dangerous and thankfully this practice has fallen out of use.

5. **C** The pentose phosphate pathway is used to generate nucleotide precursors for DNA synthesis and is therefore most active during the S phase of the cell cycle, not the M phase (choice C is a false statement and the correct answer choice). An increase in $NADP^+$, corresponding to a decrease in the $NADPH:NADP^+$ ratio, will activate the pentose phosphate pathway (choice A is true and can be eliminated). The pentose phosphate pathway (PPP) also creates NADPH, which is used as reducing power in fatty acid synthesis and also to limit oxidative stress; we would expect it to be upregulated during fatty acid synthesis (choice B is true and can be eliminated). Further, deficiencies in the PPP may increase oxidative stress in red blood cells, leading to cell lysis and hemolytic anemia (choice D is true and can be eliminated).

6. **B** Insulin levels are elevated when blood glucose levels rise, such as after consuming a large meal. Glucagon levels are elevated during fasting (choices A and C can be eliminated). Insulin allows cells to take up glucose and activates the pathways that store it as glycogen (as well as those that convert it into energy). Therefore, high insulin levels would lead to activation of the enzyme that synthesizes glycogen, glycogen synthase, and deactivation of the enzyme that breaks glycogen down, glycogen phosphorylase (choice D can be eliminated, and choice B is correct).

7. **B** The pentose phosphate pathway produces ribose, which acts as a backbone for nucleotide synthesis as well as NADPH (choice B is correct). NADH is made in catabolic reactions, such as glycolysis and the Krebs cycle (choice A is wrong). Succinyl-CoA is an intermediate product of the Krebs cycle, not the pentose phosphate pathway (choice C is wrong). Fructose-1,6-bisphosphate is one of the intermediate products of glycolysis (choice D is wrong).

SOLUTIONS TO CHAPTER 5 PRACTICE PASSAGE

1. **C** During the ischemic forearm test, blood flow is cut off from the patient's arm, reducing the delivery of oxygen to the muscles. Without oxygen, the muscle cells cannot undergo aerobic respiration and thus must undergo anaerobic respiration, producing lactate as a byproduct. Patients with GSD V have a deficiency in glycogen phosphorylase, an enzyme required to break down glycogen. As they are unable to break down glycogen, these patients will quickly consume all the glucose freely available and will not be able to produce lactic acid from anaerobic respiration (choice C is correct). Depletion of NAD^+ should not have an effect on lactate levels because NAD^+ is a byproduct of lactic acid production (the oxidation of NADH drives the reduction of pyruvate to lactate). In other words, the drop in lactic acid could explain a depletion in NAD^+, but a drop in NAD^+ cannot explain a drop in lactic acid (choice A is wrong). As glycogen cannot be broken down, the glycogen stores would also not be depleted (choice B is wrong). A drop in ADP would indicate more ATP production which is not enhanced in an ischemic state (choice D is wrong).

2. **A**   Since Item III appears in exactly two answer choices, start by evaluating it; whether it is true or false you'll be able to eliminate half the answers. Item III is false: decreased levels of glucose in the muscle cells would decrease the rate of glycolysis as well as the rate of lactic acid fermentation (choices B and D can be eliminated). Since both remaining answer choices include Item I it must be true and you can evaluate Item II. Item II is false: with decreased glycogen breakdown, there will be lower levels of glucose in the muscle cells (choice C can be eliminated and choice A is correct). Note that Item I is in fact true: because patients with GSD V lack glycogen phosphorylase, they are unable to regularly break down glycogen into glucose. As a result, these patients are expected to have elevated levels of glycogen.

3. **A**   The passage indicates that the purpose of the ischemic forearm test is to monitor levels of lactate and ammonia following exercise to confirm the diagnosis of McArdle's disease. In order to promote the production of lactate, anaerobic conditions must be favored. Without blood flow, limited oxygen will reach the forearm, creating the anaerobic environment necessary for this test (choice A is correct). Although decreased blood flow to the forearm will decrease its blood pressure, decreasing the blood pressure does not help in the diagnosis of McArdle's disease (choice B is incorrect). Generally, glycogen is not delivered to muscle via the bloodstream, but it is rather generated via glycogenesis in the muscle itself (choice C is incorrect). Preventing blood flow to the forearm may lead to decreased delivery of lactate from other parts of the body, but the purpose of stopping blood flow is to encourage the production of lactic acid, not decrease the level of lactic acid in the forearm (choice D is incorrect).

4. **D**   Patients with GSD V lack a crucial enzyme needed for glycogenolysis. As a result, these patients would exhibit decreased glycogenolysis, and glucose levels would drop. This would decrease the rate of glycolysis and lactic acid fermentation and decrease the levels of lactate in the body (choice D is correct, and choice A is wrong). Although glycogenesis may be decreased in individuals with GSD V due to the presence of excess glycogen stores, this would not be expected to substantially affect ammonia levels (choice C is wrong). In fact, the increased ammonia levels in patients with GSD V following the ischemic forearm test is primarily due to the increased breakdown of amino acids for fuel as the muscle fatigues (choice B is wrong).

5. **A**   The question stem states that under standard conditions (1 M concentration of starting materials and products), the formation of creatine phosphate is favored. Under resting conditions, ATP levels in the body are high, which favors the formation of creatine phosphate by mass action (choice A is correct, and choice C is wrong). During strenuous exercise, ATP levels drop in the body, favoring the degradation of creatine phosphate to generate more ATP (choices B and D are wrong).

Chapter 6
Lipids

The biological macromolecules are grouped into four classes of molecules that play important roles in cells and in organisms as a whole. All of them are polymers; strings of repeated units (monomers).

This chapter discusses the lipids from a biological perspective: what they are made of, how they are put together, and what their roles are in the body. These molecules are also discussed in *MCAT Organic Chemistry Review* from an organic chemistry perspective: nomenclature, chirality, etc.

6.1 INTRODUCTION TO LIPIDS

Lipids are oily or fatty substances that play three primary physiological roles, summarized here and discussed below.

1) In adipose cells, triglycerides (fats) store energy.
2) In cellular membranes, phospholipids constitute a barrier between intracellular and extracellular environments.
3) Cholesterol is a special lipid that serves as the building block for the hydrophobic steroid hormones.

The cardinal characteristic of the lipid is its **hydrophobicity**. *Hydrophobic* means "water-fearing." It is important to understand the significance of this. Since water is very polar, polar substances dissolve well in water; these are known as "water-loving," or **hydrophilic** substances. Carbon-carbon bonds and carbon-hydrogen bonds are nonpolar. Hence, substances that contain only carbon and hydrogen will not dissolve well in water. Here are some examples: table sugar dissolves well in water, but cooking oil floats in a layer above water or forms many tiny oil droplets when mixed with water. Cotton T-shirts become wet when exposed to water because they are made of glucose polymerized into cellulose, but a nylon jacket does not become wet because it is composed of atoms covalently bound together in a nonpolar fashion. A synonym for *hydrophobic* is **lipophilic** (which means "lipid-loving"); a synonym for *hydrophilic* is **lipophobic**. We return to these concepts below.

Fatty Acid Structure

Fatty acids are composed of long unsubstituted alkanes that end in a carboxylic acid. The chain is typically 14 to 18 carbons long, and because they are synthesized two carbons at a time from acetate, predominantly *even-numbered* fatty acids are made in human cells. A fatty acid with no carbon-carbon double bonds is said to be **saturated** with hydrogen because every carbon atom in the chain is covalently bound to the maximum number of hydrogens. **Unsaturated** fatty acids have one or more double bonds in the tail. These double bonds are almost always (Z) (or *cis*).

Saturated fatty acid

Unsaturated fatty acid

- How does the shape of an unsaturated fatty acid differ from that of a saturated fatty acid?[1]
- If fatty acids are mixed into water, how are they likely to associate with each other?[2]

---

[1] An unsaturated fatty acid is bent, or "kinked," at the *cis* double bond.

[2] The long hydrophobic chains will interact with each other to minimize contact with water, exposing the charged carboxyl group to the aqueous environment.

Figure 1 illustrates how free fatty acids interact in an aqueous solution; they form a structure called a **micelle**. The force that drives the tails into the center of the micelle is called the **hydrophobic interaction**. The hydrophobic interaction is a complex phenomenon. In general, it results from the fact that water molecules must form an orderly **solvation shell** around each hydrophobic substance. The reason is that H_2O has a dipole that "likes" to be able to share its charges with other polar molecules. A solvation shell allows for the most water-water interaction and the least water-lipid interaction. In the case of the fatty acid micelle, water forms a shell around the spherical micelle with the result being that water interacts with polar carboxylic acid head groups while hydrophobic lipid tails hide inside the sphere.

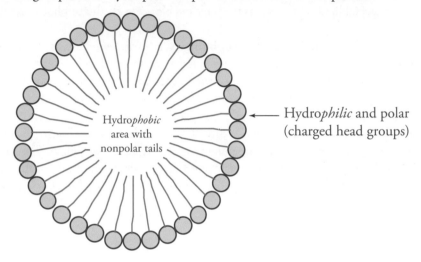

Hydro*phobic* area with nonpolar tails

← Hydro*philic* and polar (charged head groups)

Figure 1   A Fatty Acid Micelle

- How does soap help to remove grease from your hands?[3]

6.2   TRIACYLGLYCEROLS (TG)

The storage form of the fatty acid is fat. The technical name for fat is **triacylglycerol** or **triglyceride** (see Figure 2). The triglyceride is composed of three fatty acids esterified to a glycerol molecule. Glycerol is a three-carbon triol with the formula $HOCH_2–CHOH–CH_2OH$. As you can see, it has three hydroxyl groups that can be esterified to fatty acids. It is necessary to store fatty acids in the relatively inert form of fat because free fatty acids are reactive chemicals.

---

[3]   Grease is hydrophobic. It does not wash off easily in water because it is not soluble in water. Scrubbing your hands with soap causes micelles to form around the grease particles.

Figure 2 A Triglyceride (Fat)

The triacylglycerol undergoes reactions typical of esters, such as base-catalyzed hydrolysis. Soaps are the sodium salts of fatty acids ($RCOO-Na^+$). They are **amphipathic**, which means they have both hydrophilic and hydrophobic regions. Soap is economically produced by base-catalyzed hydrolysis of triglycerides from animal fat into fatty acid salts (soaps). This reaction is called **saponification** and is illustrated in Figure 3.

Triacylglycerol   Glycerol   3 Fatty Acids

Figure 3 Saponification

Lipases are enzymes that hydrolyze fats. Triacylglycerols are stored in fat cells as an energy source. Fats are more efficient energy storage molecules than carbohydrates for two reasons: packing and energy content.

1) **Packing:** Their hydrophobicity allows fats to pack together much more closely than carbohydrates. Carbohydrates carry a great amount of water-of-solvation (water molecules hydrogen-bonded to their hydroxyl groups). In other words, the amount of carbon per unit area or unit weight is much greater in a fat droplet than in dissolved sugar. If we could store sugars in a dry powdery form in our bodies, this problem would be obviated.

2) **Energy content:** All packing considerations aside, fat molecules store much more energy than carbohydrates. In other words, regardless of what you dissolve it in, a fat has more energy carbon-for-carbon than a carbohydrate. The reason is that fats are much more reduced. Remember that energy metabolism begins with the oxidation of foodstuffs to release energy. Since carbohydrates are more oxidized to start with, oxidizing them releases less energy. Animals use fat to store most of their energy, storing only a small amount as carbohydrates (glycogen). Plants such as potatoes commonly store a large percentage of their energy as carbohydrates (starch).

6.3   PHOSPHOLIPIDS AND LIPID BILAYER MEMBRANES

Membrane lipids are **phospholipids** (also called phosphatides) derived from diacylglycerol phosphate or DG-P. Often the phosphate group has even bigger polar molecules attached to it, such as choline (phosphatidylcholine), ethanolamine (phosphatidylethanolamine), and inositol (phosphatidylinositol). For example, phosphatidylcholine is a phospholipid formed by the esterification of a choline molecule $[HO(CH_2)_2N^+(CH_3)_3]$ to the phosphate group of DG-P. Phosphatidylcholine and phosphatidylethanolamine are the most common phospholipids in eukaryotic cells. Beyond its role as a membrane lipid, phosphatidylcholine is a major lipid component of lung surfactant (important in reducing surface tension inside lung alveoli), and phosphatidylinositol plays a role in signal transmission across cell membranes.

Figure 4   A Phosphoglyceride (Diacylglycerol Phosphate, or DG-P)

We saw above how fatty acids spontaneously form micelles. Phospholipids also minimize their interactions with water by forming an orderly structure—in this case, it is a **lipid bilayer** (Figure 5). Hydrophobic interactions drive the formation of the bilayer, and once formed, it is stabilized by van der Waals forces between the long tails.

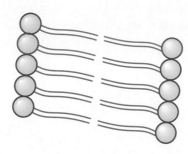

Figure 5   A Small Section of a Lipid Bilayer Membrane

- Would a saturated or an unsaturated fatty acid residue have more van der Waals interactions with neighboring alkyl chains in a bilayer membrane?[4]

A more precise way to give the answer to the question above is to say that double bonds (unsaturation) in phospholipid fatty acids *tend to increase membrane fluidity*. Unsaturation prevents the membrane from solidifying by disrupting the orderly packing of the hydrophobic lipid tails. The right amount of fluidity is essential for function. Decreasing the *length* of fatty acid tails also increases fluidity. The steroid **cholesterol** (discussed a bit later) is a third important modulator of membrane fluidity. At low temperatures, it increases fluidity in the same way as kinks in fatty acid tails; hence, it is known as *membrane antifreeze*. At high temperatures, however, cholesterol attenuates (reduces) membrane fluidity. Don't ponder this paradox too long; just remember that cholesterol keeps fluidity at an *optimum level*. Remember, the structural determinants of membrane fluidity are degree of saturation, tail length, and amount of cholesterol.

The lipid bilayer acts like a barrier surrounding the cell in the sense that it separates the interior of the cell from the exterior. However, the cell membrane is much more complex than a simple barrier; it is a dynamic structure that regulates what comes into and goes out of the cell and transmits extracellular signals to the interior of the cell. Proteins embedded in the plasma membrane play a big role in this. Since the plasma bilayer membrane surrounding cells is impermeable to charged particles such as Na^+, protein gateways such as ion channels are required for ions to enter or exit cells. Further, certain hormones (peptides) cannot pass through the cell membrane due to their charged nature; instead, protein **receptors** in the cell membrane bind these hormones and transmit a signal into the cell in a **second messenger cascade** (see *MCAT Biology Review* for more details about the plasma membrane).

6.4   TERPENES AND STEROIDS

A terpene is a member of a broad class of compounds built from isoprene units (C_5H_8) with a general formula $(C_5H_8)_n$.

Figure 6   Isoprene Unit

---

[4]   The bent shape of the unsaturated fatty acid means that it doesn't fit in as well and has less contact with neighboring groups to form van der Waals interactions. Phospholipids composed of saturated fatty acids make the membrane less fluid.

Terpenes may be linear or cyclic, and they are classified by the number of isoprene units they contain. For example, monoterpenes consist of two isoprene units, sesquiterpenes consist of three, and diterpenes contain four.

limonene
$C_{10}H_{16}$
(a monoterpene)

humulene
$C_{15}H_{24}$
(a sesquiterpene)

taxadiene
$C_{20}H_{32}$
(a diterpene)

Figure 7 Terpene Structures

Squalene is a triterpene (made of six isoprene units), and it is a particularly important compound, as it is biosynthetically utilized in the manufacture of steroids. Squalene is also a component of earwax.

Figure 8 Squalene

Whereas a terpene is formally a simple hydrocarbon, there are a number of natural and synthetically derived species that are built from an isoprene skeleton and functionalized with other elements (O, N, S, etc.). These functionalized-terpenes are known as *terpenoids*. Vitamin A ($C_{20}H_{30}O$) is an example of a terpenoid.

Figure 9 Vitamin A

Steroids

Steroids are included here because of their hydrophobicity, and, hence, similarity to fats. Their structure is otherwise unique. All steroids have the basic tetracyclic ring system (Figure 10), based on the structure of **cholesterol**, a polycyclic amphipath. (Polycyclic means several rings, and amphipathic means displaying both hydrophilic and hydrophobic characteristics.)

As discussed earlier, the steroid cholesterol is an important component of the lipid bilayer. It is both obtained from the diet and synthesized in the liver. It is carried in the blood packaged with fats and proteins into **lipoproteins**. One type of lipoprotein has been implicated as the cause of atherosclerotic vascular disease, which refers to the build-up of cholesterol "plaques" on the inside of blood vessels.

Figure 10   Cholesterol-Derived Hormones

Steroid hormones are made from cholesterol. Two examples are **testosterone** (an androgen, or male sex hormone) and **estradiol** (an estrogen, or female sex hormone). There are no receptors for steroid hormones on the surface of cells; because steroids are highly hydrophobic, they can diffuse right through the lipid bilayer membrane into the cytoplasm. The receptors for steroid hormones are located within cells rather than on the cell surface. This is an important point! You must be aware of the contrast between *peptide* hormones, such as insulin, which exert their effects by binding to receptors at the cell-surface, and *steroid* hormones, such as estrogen, which diffuse into cells to find their receptors.

6.5 OTHER LIPIDS

Beyond fatty acids, triglycerides, phospholipids, terpenes, cholesterol, and steroids, there are a few other lipids with which you should be familiar for the MCAT.

Sphingolipids

Sphingolipids are structured in a similar manner as phospholipids, except that the backbone is sphingosine instead of glycerol. The only significant sphingolipid in humans is sphingomyelin, an important component of the myelin sheath around neurons.

Figure 11   Sphingolipids

Waxes

Waxes are long chain fats esterified to long chain alcohols. They are extremely hydrophobic and often form waterproof barriers, most notably in plants. Animals also use waxes to form a protective barrier (e.g., earwax).

Figure 12 Wax

Fat-Soluble Vitamins

Fat-soluble vitamins are absorbed with dietary fat and stored in adipose tissue and in the liver. The four fat-soluble vitamins are vitamins A, D, E, and K; all of them have ring structures. Vitamin A is a terpenoid (mentioned earlier) essential for vision, growth, epithelial maintenance, and immune function. Vitamin D is derived from cholesterol (it is a steroid) important in regulating blood levels of calcium and phosphate. Vitamin E is actually a group of compounds, called **tocopherols** (methylated phenols), that are important as antioxidants. α-Tocopherol is the most active vitamin E. Vitamin K serves as an important coenzyme in the activation of clotting proteins.

Figure 13 Fat-Soluble Vitamins

Prostaglandins

Prostaglandins belong to a group of molecules known as eicosanoids, derived from 20-carbon fatty acids (the prefix *eicosa* means "20"). They have vastly different roles in different tissues, depending on the receptor to which they bind. Their roles include regulating smooth muscle contraction in the intestines and uterus, regulating blood vessel diameter, maintaining gastric integrity (by decreasing acid secretion and increasing mucus secretion), among others. They all have the same general structure, including a five-membered ring. See Figure 14.

Figure 14   Prostaglandins

6.6 FATTY ACID METABOLISM

Fatty Acid Oxidation

Following the initial steps in fat digestion, **chylomicrons** composed of fat and lipoprotein are transported via the lymphatic system and bloodstream to the liver, heart, lungs, and other organs. This dietary fat, or triacylglycerol, is then hydrolyzed to liberate free fatty acids which can then undergo β-**oxidation**. This process begins at the outer mitochondrial membrane with the activation of the fatty acid. This reaction, catalyzed by **acyl-CoA synthetase,** requires the investment of two ATP equivalents to generate a fatty acyl-CoA which is then transported into the mitochondrion.

Figure 15   Fatty Acid Activation

Once in the matrix, the fatty acyl-CoA undergoes a repeated series of four reactions which cleave the bond between the alpha and beta carbons to liberate an acetyl-CoA in addition to generating one $FADH_2$ and NADH.

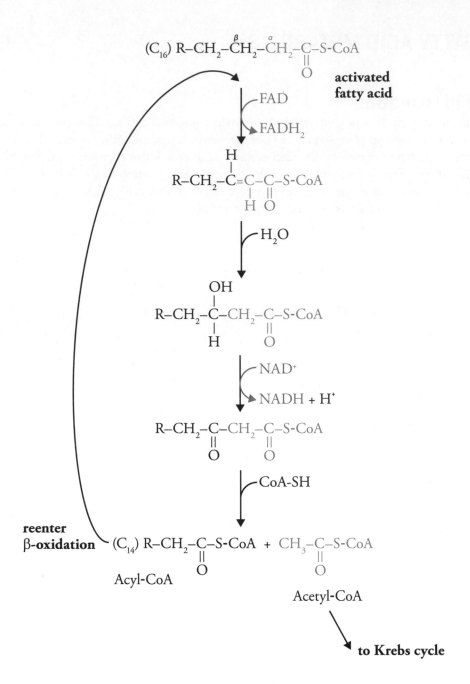

Figure 16   Fatty Acid (β) Oxidation

Each round of β-oxidation cleaves a two-carbon acetyl-CoA from the molecule; however, the final round cleaves a four-carbon fatty acyl-CoA to generate two acetyl-CoA. For instance, the complete β-oxidation of lauric acid (a 12-carbon saturated fatty acid) involves the following: an investment of two ATP equivalents to convert it to a fatty acyl-CoA and then *five* rounds of β-oxidation. This generates five $FADH_2$, five NADH, and *six* acetyl-CoA which can then enter the Krebs cycle. When these six acetyl-CoA go through the Krebs cycle, they will generate an additional 18 NADH, 6 $FADH_2$, and 6 GTP. We then have a grand total of 11 $FADH_2$ (five from β-oxidation and six from the Krebs cycle), 23 NADH (five from β-oxidation and 18 from the Krebs cycle), and six ATP equivalents (from the Krebs cycle). After the electron transport chain (and subtracting the two ATP equivalents required at the beginning of β-oxidation), we obtain 78 ATP from lauric acid.

The oxidation of unsaturated fatty acids (those containing double bonds) requires additional steps. For a monounsaturated fatty acid, β-oxidation proceeds normally, cleaving two-carbon subunits from the fatty acid, until the double bond is encountered. An isomerase then moves the double bond (if necessary) and allows the fatty acid to continue in its oxidation. If the fatty acid contains several double bonds, both the isomerase and a reductase are required to allow the fatty acid to continue through β-oxidation.

Ketogenesis

During periods of starvation, glycogen stores become exhausted and blood glucose falls significantly. To help supply the central nervous system with energy when glucose is in short supply, the liver generates **ketone bodies** via a process in the mitochondrial matrix known as **ketogenesis**. The ketone bodies are generated from acetyl-CoA and include acetone, acetoacetate, and β-hydroxybutyrate. These molecules can cross the blood-brain barrier and be converted back to acetyl-CoA once they arrive at their target organ; the acetyl-CoA can then enter the Krebs cycle (see Figure 17).

6.6

Figure 17 Ketogenesis

In some circumstances, ketogenesis can take place when adequate glucose is present in the blood but cannot enter the cell. This can occur, for example, when a patient suffering from type I diabetes does not receive an insulin injection for a prolonged period of time. Without insulin, glucose cannot enter cells in order to be used for energy, and the patient relies exclusively on fatty acid oxidation for the acetyl-CoA to turn the Krebs cycle. However, because the levels of acetyl-CoA are so high, many of them get converted into ketone bodies. Ketone bodies are acidic, and this can result in diabetic ketoacidosis, which is a potentially life-threatening condition. Patients commonly experience fatigue, confusion, and fruity-scented breath due to the acetone (which is very volatile) present in their blood. This combination of symptoms has even led to patients being mistakenly classified as intoxicated and arrested for driving under the influence.

Fatty Acid Synthesis

The *de novo* synthesis of fatty acids is reminiscent of β-oxidation with several notable exceptions. While fatty acid catabolism occurs in the mitochondrial matrix, anabolism takes place in the cytoplasm. This compartmentalization allows for easier regulation, since the enzymes required for synthesis and breakdown are separated. Much as β-oxidation involved the removal of two-carbon subunits from a fatty acid chain, the synthesis of a fatty acid involves the repeated addition of two-carbon subunits. Rather than building the nascent fatty acid directly with acetyl-CoA, acetyl-CoA is first activated in a carboxylation reaction. The activation is the committed step in fatty acid synthesis and requires the investment of ATP; it is facilitated by **acetyl-CoA carboxylase** to generate **malonyl-CoA**.

Figure 18   Synthesis of Malonyl-CoA

Fatty acid synthase is a large enzyme with multiple catalytic domains. Acetyl-CoA first binds to a domain known as the **acyl carrier protein (ACP)**. It is then shifted to another domain on the enzyme with a cysteine residue, and malonyl-CoA binds to the ACP. The acetyl group condenses with the malonyl group as the malonyl is decarboxylated. (Recall that the successive addition, then removal of CO_2 can drive unfavorable reactions; this same process occurs in gluconeogenesis with the carboxylation of pyruvate to oxaloacetate, and the subsequent decarboxylation of oxaloacetate to PEP.) The ACP domain now holds a four-carbon unit, which undergoes two reductions. This process requires the reducing power of NADPH, which is generally obtained from the pentose phosphate pathway (see Chapter 5). The saturated four-carbon acyl unit is shifted to the domain with the cysteine residue, and another malonyl-CoA binds to the ACP. The process then repeats: the four-carbon unit condenses with malonyl as CO_2 is lost, two successive reductions occur, and the now six-carbon chain is shifted to the cysteine residue.

6.6

Figure 19 Fatty Acid Synthesis

Once a 16-carbon long fatty acid is generated, additional enzymes aid in further modification of the fatty acid (e.g., addition of functional groups and elongation). Note that this process requires no template (nor does glycogen or amino acid synthesis), which means that nothing is "read" to generate the products. This differs from the template-based syntheses of polypeptides (mRNA is "read" to generate an amino acid sequence) and nucleic acids (DNA is "read" to generate DNA during replication and RNA during transcription; for more information on these processes, see *MCAT Biology Review*).

6.7 AMINO ACID CATABOLISM AND METABOLIC SUMMARY

We discussed amino acid structure and protein structure and function in Chapter 4, but we haven't yet really touched on the idea of proteins as fuel. Proteins in cells are constantly being made, kept for a certain period of time (minutes to weeks), and then degraded back into amino acids. In addition, humans absorb amino acids from dietary proteins. These free amino acids can be catabolized via several pathways. They can be taken up by cells and used to make cellular proteins. The amino group can be removed and either used to synthesize nitrogenous compounds, such as nucleotide bases, or it can be converted into urea for excretion. The remaining carbon skeleton (also called an α-keto acid) can either be broken down into water and CO_2, or it can be converted to glucose (glucogenic amino acids) or acetyl-CoA (ketogenic amino acids).

Figure 20 Protein Breakdown

Metabolism Summary

Generally speaking, cells prefer to use carbohydrates as fuel. When blood sugar is high, cells will take up glucose and make ATP via glycolysis. Liver and muscle cells will also store glucose as glycogen (glycogenesis), and the liver can also take some of the acetyl-CoA generated by the pyruvate dehydrogenase complex to make fatty acids (fatty acid synthesis). These are converted into triglycerides and stored in adipose tissue. These pathways are shown in black in Figure 21.

When blood sugar levels fall (starved state), the liver will break down the stored glycogen (glycogenolysis) and release glucose into the bloodstream. It will also begin the process of gluconeogenesis to synthesize "new" glucose that can also be released into the bloodstream. This glucose can be taken up by other body cells and used in glycolysis to generate ATP. These pathways are shown in green in Figure 21.

6.7

If the starved state continues past the point at which all glycogen stores are used (12–24 hours), then fatty acid breakdown will occur. Triglycerides from adipose tissue are broken down into free fatty acids and glycerol that are released into the bloodstream. Cells will take up the fatty acids and run β-oxidation. The liver can use the glycerol to generate glucose in gluconeogenesis. Some of the acetyl-CoA made in β-oxidation is used to turn the Krebs cycle, and some is converted into ketone bodies (ketogenesis). These pathways are shown in red in Figure 21.

Finally, proteins and amino acids can be used as fuel. The carbon skeleton of the amino acids can be used in gluconeogenesis (glucogenic amino acids) or to make acetyl-CoA and ketone bodies (ketogenic amino acids).

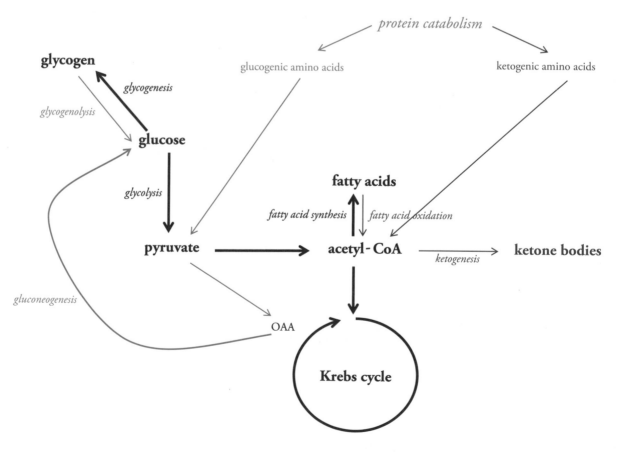

Figure 21   Summary of Metabolism

Chapter 6 Summary

- Lipids are found in several forms in the body, including (but not limited to) triglycerides, phospholipids, cholesterol and steroids, and terpenes. Triglycerides and phospholipids are linear, while cholesterol and steroids have a ring structure.

- Lipids are hydrophobic. Triglycerides are used for energy storage, phospholipids form membranes, and cholesterol is the precursor to the steroid hormones.

- Other lipids include sphingolipids, waxes, fat-soluble vitamins, and prostaglandins.

- The only significant sphingolipid is sphingomyelin, found in the myelin sheath of neurons.

- Waxes are long-chain fats esterified to long-chain alcohols and act as very hydrophobic protective barriers.

- Fat-soluble vitamins include vitamins A, D, E, and K. Vitamin A is necessary for vision, vitamin D is essential for bone structure and calcium regulation, vitamin E is an antioxidant, and vitamin K is important for blood clotting.

- Fatty acid (or beta) oxidation is the repetitive removal of 2-carbon units as acetyl-CoA from the fatty acid. Each round of fatty acid oxidation yields 1 $FADH_2$ and 1 NADH. The acetyl units can enter the Krebs cycle or be converted to ketone bodies.

- Fatty acid synthesis requires high amounts of ATP and NADPH. Fats are synthesized by the successive addition of 2-carbon units to the fatty acid chain until a 16-carbon fat is produced.

- During starvation, acetyl-CoA from fatty acid oxidation can be converted into ketone bodies (acetone, acetoacetate, and β-hydroxybutyrate). The ketone bodies can easily travel through the blood and supply energy to the brain (all can be reconverted to acetyl-CoA), but can also lower blood pH.

- When the body is in a well-fed state (e.g., blood glucose levels are high), glycolysis, glycogenesis, and fatty acid synthesis are favored. When the body is in a starved state (e.g., blood glucose levels are low), glycogenolysis, gluconeogenesis, and fatty acid oxidation are favored.

CHAPTER 6 FREESTANDING PRACTICE QUESTIONS

1. Which property of lipids contributes most to their higher energy density per carbon in comparison to carbohydrates?

A) Lipids can contain more double bonds in existing carbon chains than carbohydrates can in cyclic structures.
B) Carbohydrates exist in a more oxidized state, while lipids are more reduced.
C) Carbohydrates are absorbed more easily than lipids by the digestive system.
D) Lipids can contribute more isoprenes to the Krebs cycle than carbohydrates.

2. Artemisinin, a drug used as part of a multi-valent approach to treating malaria, is a sesquiterpene now being produced in yeast. The biosynthesis of sesquiterpenes requires how many isoprene units?

A) 1
B) 2
C) 3
D) 4

3. Fatty acid synthesis requires all of the following EXCEPT:

I. ACP
II. ADP
III. NADPH

A) I only
B) II only
C) I and III only
D) II and III only

4. An inhibitor of isomerases in fatty acid oxidation would most hinder the catabolism of:

A) terpenes.
B) saturated fatty acids.
C) phospholipids.
D) unsaturated fatty acids.

5. Increasing the amount of cholesterol in a plasma membrane would lead to an increase in:

A) permeability.
B) atherosclerotic plaques.
C) melting temperature.
D) freezing temperature.

6. Stearic acid is a 16-carbon saturated fatty acid. Including those made in the Krebs cycle, how many NADH and $FADH_2$ would be produced by the complete oxidation of stearic acid?

A) 15 $FADH_2$ and 15 NADH
B) 16 $FADH_2$ and 16 NADH
C) 15 $FADH_2$ and 31 NADH
D) 16 $FADH_2$ and 32 NADH

CHAPTER 6 PRACTICE PASSAGE

Some lipid molecules in the plasma membrane display asymmetry in membrane distribution. For example, glycolipids are found exclusively in the noncytosolic side of the lipid bilayer. This means that the cell surface is covered in carbohydrates, which can be covalently linked to other biological macromolecules. The plasma membrane can contain glycoproteins, glycosaminoglycans, and glycosphingolipids (GSLs).

GSLs consist of a lipid molecule called *ceramide*, linked to carbohydrates; this is a diverse group of macromolecules with over 300 members. The diversity hinges on the carbohydrate chains and variation in glycan buildup. Catalysis of glycan addition is directed by a range of proteins involved in biosynthesis. Of this enzyme family, glycosyltransferases are well studied and the mechanism of action for many glycosyltransferase enzymes has been determined and published.

Glycolipids tend to associate together in the plasma membranes, forming microdomains and lipid rafts. These associations are likely to facilitate glycolipid function, which can include immune cell development, protection of the cell against harsh conditions, facilitating cell to cell interactions, maintaining plasma membrane integrity, cell signaling, and membrane transport.

Globotriaosylceramide (GL3) is a glycosphingolipid and is formed by alpha linkage of galactose to lactosylceramide. Biosynthesis of lactosylceramide includes expansion of the monosaccharide chain by adding a galactose unit to monoglucosylceramide. Lactosylceramide is found in small amounts in most tissues. In contrast, ceramides are found in high concentrations within the cell membrane of most eukaryotic cells. A ceramide is composed of sphingosine and a fatty acid. A recent study examined the levels of GL3 in specific human cell types (Figure 1). Four biopsies of metastatic cancers were also tested for GL3 levels (Figure 2).

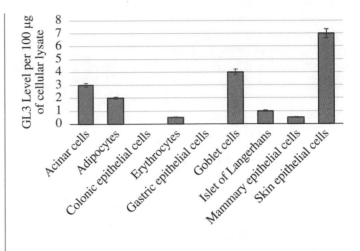

Figure 1 GL3 levels in some human cell types

Figure 2 GL3 levels in metastatic cancer biopsy samples

1. Which of the following is true of glycosyltransferases?

A) They function in the Golgi apparatus and transfer carbohydrate groups to lipid molecules.
B) These enzymes are made of ceramide linked to carbohydrates.
C) They function outside the cell and transfer carbohydrate groups to lipid molecules.
D) They are enzymes and proteins, but their mechanism of action is unknown.

2. Accumulation of GL3 has been implicated in a metabolic disease. Which of the following would be the best way to inhibit this accumulation?

A) Activation of lactosylceramide 4-α-galactosyltransferase, which synthesizes globotriaosylceramide.
B) Activation of β-1,4-galactosyltransferase, which synthesizes lactosylceramide.
C) Activation of α-galactosidase, which degrades globotriaosylceramide.
D) Competitive inhibition of α-galactosidase, which degrades globotriaosylceramide.

3. Globotriaosylsphingosine (lyso-Gb3) is a GL3 metabolite and could be a promising secondary screening biomarker for:

   I. colon cancer.
   II. skin cancer.
   III. stomach cancer.

A) I only
B) II and III only
C) I and III only
D) I, II, and III

4. Based on the known functions of glycolipids, which of the following can be inferred?

A) Glycolipids associate with other biological macromolecules, such as proteins.
B) Glycolipids are isolated in lipid rafts and do not associate with proteins.
C) Lipids rafts are made of protein clusters and do not include lipids.
D) At least 30% of human cells must express appreciable levels of glycolipids.

5. Based on the data presented in the passage, all of the following are true EXCEPT:

A) expression of GL3 in colonic epithelial cells is a good indicator that the cells have become cancerous.
B) since it is expressed in all four types of metastatic cancer cells, GL3 is a good screening marker for all four types of metastatic cancer.
C) the expression of GL3 in stomach cancer cells is a better indicator that the cells might metastasize than the expression of GL3 in breast cancer cells.
D) there is a significant difference in the expression of GL3 between goblet cells and acinar cells.

6. Globotriaosylceramide contains:

A) two monosaccharides linked to the intracellular side of a ceramide lipid in the plasma membrane
B) two monosaccharides linked to the extracellular side of a ceramide lipid in the plasma membrane
C) three monosaccharides linked to the intracellular side of a ceramide lipid in the plasma membrane
D) three monosaccharides linked to the extracellular side of a ceramide lipid in the plasma membrane

SOLUTIONS TO CHAPTER 6 FREESTANDING PRACTICE QUESTIONS

1. **B** Energy production in cells is essentially based on oxidation. Since carbohydrates are more oxidized per carbon and lipids are more reduced, the catabolism of lipids can produce more energy (choice B is correct). While an unsaturated fatty acid would have double bonds, this does not address the question of why, on a per-carbon basis, lipids in general yield more energy than carbohydrates (choice A is wrong). The ease of absorption has nothing to do with energy density per carbon (choice C is wrong). Isoprenes are not utilized by the Krebs cycle (choice D is wrong).

2. **C** The prefix *sesqui-* means "one and a half," so a sesquiterpene is made up of one and a half terpenes. A terpene is at minimum two isoprene units, so a sesquiterpene, one and a half terpenes, would be made up of three isoprene units (choice C is correct). One isoprene unit creates to a hemiterpene (half a terpene; choice A is wrong), two isoprene units creates a monoterpene (choice B is wrong), and four isoprene units creates a diterpene (choice D is wrong).

3. **B** Item I is false: ACP, acyl-carrier protein, is a subunit of the fatty acid synthase enzyme and replaces coenzyme A on both acetyl-CoA and malonyl-CoA as part of the activation steps of fatty acid synthesis (ACP is required for fatty acid synthesis, so choices A and C can be eliminated). Since both of the remaining choices include Item II, it must be true and we can go directly to Item III. Item III is false: NADPH is used during the elongation steps of fatty acid synthesis as reducing power (NADPH is required for fatty acid synthesis; choice D can be eliminated, and choice B is correct). Note that Item II is true: ADP is not used in fatty acid synthesis. Instead, ATP is needed to convert acetyl-CoA and bicarbonate into malonyl-CoA. Of the three given items, ADP is the only one not required for fatty acid synthesis.

4. **D** Isomerases are used during β-oxidation of unsaturated fatty acids to ensure correct placement of a carbon-carbon double bond for the process to begin (choice D is correct). Terpenes are specialized fats (such as squalene) and phospholipids are membrane lipids, neither of which go through β-oxidation (choices A and C are wrong), and the β-oxidation of saturated fats does not require isomerase (choice B is wrong).

5. **C** Plasma membranes can be up to 50% composed of sterols. Sterols help stabilize the membrane at both spectrums of the temperature. At low temperatures, they increase fluidity because the ring structure of cholesterol does not allow for tight phospholipid tail packing. This decreases the temperature at which the membrane would freeze (choice D is wrong). At high temperatures, cholesterol decreases membrane fluidity (the OH group of cholesterol prevents phospholipid dispersion) and permeability (by filling in the "holes" between the fatty acid tails; choice A is wrong), thus increasing the temperature at which membranes would melt (choice C is correct). The formation of atherosclerotic plaques, while related to cholesterol, is due to high levels of blood cholesterol, not membrane cholesterol (choice B is wrong).

6. **C** A 16-carbon fatty acid will require 7 turns of β-oxidation to produce 8 acetyl CoA, which will subsequently go through the Krebs cycle. Each turn of the β-oxidation cycle produces 1 $FADH_2$ and 1 NADH, and each turn of the Krebs cycle produces 1 $FADH_2$ and 3 NADH. 7 $FADH_2$ + 7 NADH + 8 $FADH_2$ + 24 NADH = 15 $FADH_2$ and 31 NADH (choice C is correct, and choices A, B, and D are wrong).

SOLUTIONS TO CHAPTER 6 PRACTICE PASSAGE

1. **A** According to the passage, glycosyltransferases are enzymes that catalyze the addition of sugar groups to lipids. Most enzymes are proteins, and so are made of amino acids (eliminate choice B). The passage also says glycosyltransferases are well studied and the mechanism of action for many glycosyltransferase enzymes has been determined and published (eliminate choice D). This leaves options A and C as the potential answer. These answer choices differ in where glycosyltransferases function. While the carbohydrate portions of glycolipids are found on the extracellular surface of the plasma membrane, there is no information in the passage to support that glycosyltransferases function outside of the cell (eliminate choice C). The Golgi apparatus is involved in macromolecule trafficking to the plasma membrane and contains enzymes that modify carbohydrate groups on many macromolecules. It is more likely that glycosyltransferases function in the Golgi apparatus than outside the cell (choice A is correct).

2. **C** The question stem tells you that GL3 accumulation is causing a metabolic disease. The best treatment for this disease would be one that blocks or inhibits this accumulation. Activation of the enzyme that synthesizes GL3 would lead to even more GL3; this is the opposite of what you're looking for (eliminate choice A). Lactosylceramide is a building block of GL3. Activating the enzyme that makes lactosylceramide would not decrease GL3 levels (eliminate choice B). Both choices C and D discuss the enzyme that catabolizes (or breaks down) GL3. A good way to decrease GL3 accumulation would be to activate the enzyme that breaks it down; competitive inhibition of that enzyme would reduce its function (eliminate choice D, choice C is correct).

3. **C** Since this is a Roman numeral question, start by analyzing the item that appears in exactly two answer choices; whether it is true or false you'll be able to eliminate half the answers. In this case, Item II is found in exactly two choices. Item II is false: first, from the information in the question stem, lyso-Gb3 is a metabolite of GL3. This means that if a tissue type has high GL3, it may have high lyso-Gb3 as well. Based on Figure 2, skin cancer cells express GL3, but from Figure 1, so do normal skin cells, and at the same level of skin cancer cells. Thus, lyso-Gb3 is not a good secondary screening biomarker for skin cancer (choices B and D can be eliminated). Since both remaining choices include Item I it must be true and we can focus on Item III. Item III is true: stomach cancer cells express some GL3 (Figure 2), but normal stomach (gastric) epithelial cells do not (Figure 1), so lyso-Gb3 could be a good secondary screening marker for stomach cancer (choice A can be eliminated and choice C is correct). Note that Item I is in fact true: similar to stomach cancer cells, colon cancer cells express GL3 at high levels (Figure 2), but normal colon epithelial cells do not (Figure 1), so lyso-Gb3 could be a good secondary screening marker for colon cancer.

4. **A** The passage says that glycolipids function in cell signaling and membrane transport. Based on this, it is highly likely they associate and cooperate with membrane proteins (choice A is correct; eliminate choice B). The passage says that lipid rafts contain glycolipids (eliminate choice C). There is no way to know if answer choice D is true or not based on information in the passage. This very specific statement is not supported (eliminate choice D).

5. **B**   Make sure to highlight the word "EXCEPT" and write "A B C D" on your noteboard. Evaluate each answer choice, writing "T" if it is true and "F" if it is false. Since GL3 is expressed at a very high level in metastatic colonic cancer cells, and not at all in normal colonic cells, the expression of GL3 is a good indicator of colon cancer (write "T" next to "A" on the noteboard). Although GL3 is expressed in all four types of cancer, the level of expression in breast cancer cells and skin cancer cells is exactly the same as the level of expression in normal mammary and skin cells. While GL3 might be a good screening marker for colon and stomach cancer, it would likely not be a good screening marker for breast and skin cancer (write "F" next to "B" on the noteboard). Similar to choice A, metastatic stomach cancer cells express GL3 at a much higher level than normal gastric cells, while breast cancer cells and normal mammary cells express GL3 at the same level. While breast cancer cells can still metastasize (and do), the presence of GL3 in those cells is not as good an indicator of the likelihood for metastasis as the presence of GL3 in stomach cancer cells (write "T" next to "C" on the noteboard). Both goblet cells and acinar cells express GL3, with goblet cells having a higher level of expression than acinar cells. Since the error bars do not overlap for these two cell types, it can be said that the difference in expression is significant (write "T" next to "D" on the noteboard). Since choice B stands out with an "F" instead of a "T," it the correct answer choice.

6. **D**   The passage says that the carbohydrate groups of glycolipids are expressed on the extracellular surface of the cell (eliminate choices A and C). The last paragraph of the passage says that a fatty acid and a sphingosine join to form a ceramide. A glucose is added to form monoglucosylceramide. A galactose is added to form lactosylceramide. Another galactose is added to form globotriaosylceramide. This means that GL3 is made of a ceramide lipid with three carbohydrate groups (eliminate choice B, choice D is correct).

NEROLIDOL, A SESQUITERPENE, ATTENUATES OXIDATIVE STRESS AND INFLAMMATION IN ACETIC ACID-INDUCED COLITIS IN RATS

Salim M. A. Bastaki[1], Naheed Amir[1], Ernest Adeghate[2], Shreesh Ojha[1]

Received: 5 September 2020 / Accepted: 29 January 2021 / Published online: 17 May 2021

INTRODUCTION

Inflammatory bowel disease (IBD) is an incurable chronic intestinal disorder of the gastrointestinal (GI) tract. The principal types of IBD are ulcerative colitis and Crohn's disease (CD), which are characterized by chronic inflammation of the intestine with alternating relapses and remissions and requires long-term treatment. Although it is considered a group of complex heterogeneous gastrointestinal disease that involves genetic variations, intestinal microbiota, immunological factors, and environmental factors, which interact with an inherent genetic predisposition, the underlying mechanism remains unknown. The inappropriate immune response to environment changes and the gut microbiota are among the main causes of intestinal inflammation in IBD. Experimental models and clinical studies data suggest that oxidative signaling through multiple functional levels is the major underlying mechanism in the pathogenesis of IBD. The products of oxidative stress along with rising inflammation caused by induction and release of pro-inflammatory cytokines contribute to damages of the mucosal layer in the GI tract, bacterial invasion, which in turn triggers immune response and eventually cell death. Thus, targeting inflammation and oxidative stress represents an important therapeutic target for IBD.

The available therapies for IBD are not very satisfactory for the majority of the patients who require continuous medication to keep the disease under control. In addition, the currently used agents including aminosalicylates, corticosteroids, immunomodulators, and biological agents often elicit variable responses with side effects and a diminishing therapeutic benefit over time. Aside from radical surgery for refractory ulcerative colitis, there is no cure or preventive measures available. Various treatment strategies have been shown initially to exert beneficial effects for the treatment of IBD, but prolonged treatments resulted in severe side effects. An ideal agent would prevent relapses and maintain remission with minimal adverse effects and lesser variation in therapeutic effects.

The use of many plants in therapeutics is based on traditional consumption in diets for health benefits since ancient times. In recent years, numerous plant-derived bioactive compounds known as phytochemicals and also referred to as phytobiotics or phytogenics have raised interest for their therapeutic potential in IBD due to multiple pharmacological properties. These bioactive compounds have been shown to ameliorate intestinal inflammation through reduction of inflammatory cytokines and modulation of intracellular signaling transduction pathways. To date, many novel dietary compounds of natural origin, belonging to different classes of phytochemicals such as glycosides, alkaloids, terpenes, saponins, and flavonoids, have been shown to be effective in experimental models of colitis by targeting oxidative stress and immune-inflammatory cascade.

Among different classes, the terpenes commonly found in essential oils of edible plants have generated immense interest due to their favorable pharmacological properties and therapeutic effects in gastrointestinal diseases. One of the dietary bioactive phytochemicals, nerolidol (NRD), a naturally occurring aliphatic sesquiterpene alcohol has garnered attention for its therapeutic potential in human diseases along with its dietary and cosmetic use. It is widely present in ornamental as well as edible plants including *Oplopanax horridus* and *Thymus alternans* and has been found to be beneficial to health. It is widely

Salim M. A. Bastaki

[1] Department of Pharmacology and Therapeutics, College of Medicine and Health Sciences, United Arab Emirates University, PO Box 17666, Al Ain, Abu Dhabi, United Arab Emirates

[2] Department of Anatomy, College of Medicine and Health Sciences, United Arab Emirates University, PO Box 17666, Al Ain, Abu Dhabi, United Arab Emirates

used as flavor enhancer, in a traditional semi-oxidized Chinese tea known as Oolong tea and Portuguese Madeira wines. It has been included in the list of safe compounds by the US Food and Drug Administration (USFDA) for its use in the food industry as a preservative and flavoring agent. NRD has been shown to possess neuroprotective, hepatoprotective, cardioprotective, genoprotective, antinociceptive and wound-healing properties, which is mainly attributed to its action in reducing inflammation. Studies have shown that NRD ameliorates drug- and toxicant-induced oxidative stress and inflammatory events in body organs such as brain, kidney, liver, heart, lungs, testes, eye, stomach, and uterus. Despite the potent antioxidant and anti-inflammatory roles in various organs, there are no reports available on its role in colonic tissues to demonstrate its therapeutic potential in colitis.

NRD is a lipophilic and highly bioavailable agent that makes it able to achieve required concentration for its therapeutic effect and restores redox balance by abolishing oxidative stress and subsequent inflammatory responses involving many pathways. In a preliminary study, NRD was shown to have a protective effect against ethanol-, indomethacin-, and stress-induced gastric ulcer and to significantly inhibit ulcer formation. Additionally, NRD has been shown to inhibit cell growth and proliferation and to induce cell death in colon cancer (SW-480, and HCT-116 cells). Integrating therapeutic roles of NRD in gastric tissues and colon cancer along with its property of inhibiting ROS inflammation, it was thought worthwhile to evaluate the therapeutic eff of NRD in experimental model of colitis.

Therefore, the aim of the present study was to investigate the effect of NRD on Acetic acid (AA) induced IBD and underlying antioxidant and anti-inflammatory mechanisms in the rat model. In addition, the effects of NRD on colonic macroscopic and microscopic changes were also investigated. Furthermore, the suppression of free radical formation by the endogenous antioxidant defense system and the levels of inflammatory mediators such as cytokines and calprotectin were also measured in AA-induced IBD in rats.

MATERIALS AND METHODS

Experimental animals
Adult male albino Wistar rats weighing 225–240 g were maintained at the experimental animal research facility housed in polycarbonate cages lined with husk (replaced every 24 h), under standard laboratory conditions required for animal house viz. photoperiod of 12-h light–dark cycle, room temperature at 22 °C, and humidity at 55%. The rodent chow diet was obtained commercially and water was available to the animals ad libitum. The animals were randomly divided into different groups and acclimatized for a week before commencing the experiments. They were fasted for 24 h prior to the induction of colitis by intrarectal administration of 1 ml of 4% AA at 8 cm proximal to the anus for 30 s under the influence of light anesthesia with ether after overnight fasting. The rats were kept in Trendelenburg position during rectal instillation and for 1 min after instillation to prevent leakage of the solution. To flush the colon, 1 ml of phosphate-buffered saline (PBS) was also administered in similar conditions.

Experimental design
The dose of NRD 50 mg/kg was chosen based on a dose–response pilot study in our laboratory and the basis of results published from our labs and other previous studies on antioxidant and anti-inflammatory properties. NRD was administered under two different regimens: (1) therapeutic regimen wherein the effect of NRD was tested for 1 week after the induction of IBD and (2) prophylactic, wherein NRD was administered 3 days before the induction of IBD and continued for 7 days after IBD induction. In summary, for each treatment modality, rats were divided into pre-IBD NRD-treated (n = 18) and post-IBD NRD-treated groups (n = 18). NRD 50 mg/kg in olive oil was administered orally 30 min after the induction of IBD (post-treated groups) daily. Control animals received olive oil alone using the same technique. The animals were weighed at 0, 2, 4, and 7 days after IBD and colon samples from control and post- and pretreatment groups were collected in liquid nitrogen and 4% neutral buffered formalin.

Assessment of macroscopic ulcer score
To examine the extent of colonic inflammation by macroscopic and microscopic analysis, histological samples were collected at selected time points (0 day and after 2, 4, and 7 days of IBD with or without NRD treatment). On the 7th day after IBD, the rats were euthanized by cervical dislocation and the colons were excised 2 cm above the anal margin, opened longitudinally, and washed with saline. Macroscopic damage was assessed by a previously described and well-established scoring method, which takes into account the area of inflammation and the presence or absence of ulcers. The criteria for assessing macroscopic damage were based on a semi-quantitative scoring system where features are graded as follows: 0, no ulcer, no inflammation; 1, no ulcer, local hyperemia; 2, ulceration without hyperemia; 3, ulceration

and inflammation at one site only; 4, two or more sites of ulceration and inflammation; and 5, ulceration extending more than 2 cm.

Assessment of microscopic ulcer score

After macroscopic observation, samples of the colon were subsequently excised and processed for microscopic observation according to a previously described method.

Preparation of colon tissue homogenate

Samples of 8 cm portion of distal colon were cut longitudinally to open and washed with ice-cold PBS. The tissue was weighed and homogenized with complete protease inhibitor cocktail. The resulting homogenates, after 30 min incubation on ice, were centrifuged at 15,000 rpm for 30 min at 4 °C. The obtained supernatant was stored at −40 °C until ELISA. Protein concentration was determined in each sample by a commercially available kit following BCA method.

Determination of myeloperoxidase activity in colon

Myeloperoxidase (MPO) was measured by sandwich ELISA according to manufacturer's protocols.

Determination of calprotectin in colon

Enzyme immunoassay of calprotectin, in distal colon protein samples, was performed by using commercially available sandwich ELISA kit.

Measurements of glutathione content in colon

The glutathione (GSH) content in colon homogenate was estimated following manufacturer's protocol of the assay kit. Briefly, the kinetic assay method was used to measure in which catalytic amounts (nmoles) of GSH cause a continuous reduction of 5,5-dithiobis (2-nitrobenzoic acid) to nitrobenzoic acid (TNB), and the glutathione disulfide (GSSG) formed was recycled by glutathione reductase and NADPH.

Determination of catalase activity in colon

Catalase (CAT) activity was measured by catalase assay kit which utilized the peroxidation function of CAT for determination of enzyme activity. The method was based on the reaction of the enzyme with methanol in the presence of an optimal concentration of H_2O_2. The formaldehyde produced was measured spectrophotometrically.

Determination of superoxide dismutase (SOD) in colon

Superoxide dismutase (SOD) activity was determined by SOD assay kit following the manufacturer's protocol. This colorimetric assay utilized the tetrazolium salt for detection of superoxide radicals generated by xanthine oxidase and hypoxanthine.

Measurement of malondialdehyde

The lipid peroxidation product, malondialdehyde (MDA), in the colon homogenate from each group, was measured using MDA assay kit. The assay is based on the reaction of MDA with thiobarbituric acid (TBA) to form an adduct MDA-TBA that absorbs strongly at 532 nm.

Determination of Inflammatory cytokines TNF-α, IL-1β, IL-6, and IL-23 in colon

Enzyme immunoassay of TNFα, IL-1β, IL-6, and IL-23 in colon homogenate was performed by using commercial sandwich duo set ELISA kit.

Table 1   Effect of nerolidol (NRD) on body weight (g) in IBD rat model

Day	Non-IBD control	IBD control	IBD post-nerolidol-treated	Pre-IBD nerolidol-treated
Day 0	220 ± 2.00	221 ± 5.00	224 ± 6.00	216 ± 2.00
Day 2	231 ± 4.00	209 ± 3.30***	214 ± 5.00##	237 ± 4.60###
Day 4	240 ± 3.50	213 ± 5.00***	217 ± 7.00#	240 ± 4.60###
Day 7	250 ± 3.00	206 ± 3.40***	224 ± 5.00##	240 ± 4.57###

***$P< 0.001$ day 0 non IBD control group vs IBD control group; #$P< 0.05$, ##$P< 0.01$, ###$P< 0.001$, IBD control group vs post/pre-treatment

Statistical analysis

SPSS 23.0 software was used for statistical analyses of the data which are presented as mean ± standard error of mean (SEM). Independent t-test was used for data analyses and to determine the significance of the mean between the groups. Values of $P < 0.05$ were considered significant.

RESULTS

Effect of nerolidol on mean body weight (BW) in acetic acid-induced IBD

Table 1 shows the mean BW of rats treated with NRD either 3 days before or after the induction of IBD, by gastric gavage at doses of 50 mg/kg per day.   The mean BW of rats was significantly reduced by IBD ($P < 0.001$). After the induction of IBD, administration of NRD at a dose of 50 mg/kg orally and continued for 7 days, significantly ($P < 0.05$-$P<0.01$) decreased the mean BW. The mean BW of Pre-IBD NRD treated was significantly ($P < 0.001$) increased.

Effect of nerolidol on mean macroscopic ulcer score in acetic acid-induced IBD

Figures 1a and b show the effect of oral administration of NRD on macroscopic changes and mean macroscopic ulcer score (MAUS) in rats, respectively, after AA-induced IBD. The colonic mucosa of control (untreated) rats showed marked ulceration and hyperemia (Fig. 1a). After the induction of IBD, there was a significant ($P <0.001$) increase in mean MAUS (Fig. 1b). Administration of 50 mg/kg NRD produced a significant ($P <0.05$-$P <0.001$) decrease in mean MAUS when administered either 3 days before or 30 min post IBD when compared to control (IBD, untreated, $n = 6$) (Fig. 1b). Mean MAUS reduces, when compared

to control (IBD, untreated) (Fig. 1b). Similarly, when NRD was administered post-IBD, there was a significant ($P < 0.05$, $P < 0.01$, $n=6$) reduction in the mean MAUS (Fig. 1b).

Effect of nerolidol on mean microscopic ulcer score in AA-induced IBD

Figures 2a and b show the effect of oral administration of NRD on light microscopic (histological) changes and mean microscopic ulcer score (MiUS) in rats, respectively, after AA-induced IBD. There was a significant ($P < 0.001$) increase in microscopic ulcer score (MiUS) after the induction of IBD (Fig. 2b). Administration of NRD 3 days before the induction of IBD at a dose of 50 mg/kg, resulted in a non-significant reduction in MiUS on all the days tested (Fig. 2b). NRD administered orally at a dose of 50 mg/kg after the induction of IBD in rats significantly ($P < 0.05$, $P < 0.01$, $n=6$) reduced MiUS (Fig. 2b).

a: Effect of nerolidol on colon macroscopic ulcer score in acetic acid-induced IBD

Non IBD Control   2 days IBD   4 days IBD   7 days IBD

a: IBD Control (no Nerolidol); b: Post IBD Nerolidol treatment; c: Pre IBD Nerolidol treatment

Fig. 1 Effect of nerolidol on macroscopic image (a), ulcer score (b) in IBD rat model. Data are mean ± SEM. *Significant difference between nerolidol-treated and non-IBD control. #Significant difference between nerolidol-treated and IBD control. ***$P < 0.001$; #$P < 0.05$, ##$P < 0.01$, ###$P < 0.001$

Administration of NRD to rats after the induction of IBD also reduced lymphatic infiltration in the colon (Fig. 2a). Fig. 2a shows the effect of NRD on microscopic structure in the colonic mucosa of treated and untreated rats. Figures 2a-B1, 2C1, 2D1, showed a colonic mucosa which was severely inflamed and necrotic with inflammatory cell infiltration, edema, hyperemia and goblet cell hyperplasia. As shown in Fig. 2a, cross section histopathological screening of the rat's colon tissue, revealed normal looking mucosal epithelium with neither necrosis nor inflammation in the control group. Pre- (Figures 2b-B2, C2, D2) and post-treatment (Figures 2a-B3, C3, D3) with NRD resulted in healing of the mucosal epithelium, a reduction in inflammatory edema, and a reduction in necrotic tissues and eroded surfaces. Hyperemia was not observed in NRD-treated groups.

Effect of nerolidol on mean calprotectin levels in acetic acid-induced IBD

Figure 3 shows the effect of NRD treatment on calprotectin, a marker of bowel inflammation in colon tissues, administered either 3 days before or 30 min after the induction of IBD in rats and continued for 7 days. There was a significant ($P < 0.01$, $P < 0.001$, $n = 6$) increase in calprotectin levels 2 and 7 days after the induction of IBD. Colonic calprotectin levels were unaffected after 4 days of IBD. Administration of NRD, 30 min after the induction of IBD significantly ($P < 0.001$, $n=6$) decreased colon calprotectin levels on days 2 of IBD, but was non-significant on days 4 and 7 of IBD. Administration of NRD 3 days before the induction of IBD, caused significant ($P < 0.05$, $P < 0.01$, $n = 6$) reduction in colonic calprotectin levels on days 2 and 7 of IBD. Colonic calprotectin levels were unaffected by NRD after 4 days of IBD.

Effect of nerolidol on mean glutathione levels in acetic acid-induced IBD

Fig. 4a shows the effect of NRD on mean colonic tissue levels of glutathione (GSH) in rats. GSH in control (no IBD, no NRD) was 35.50 ± 3.66 μM ($n = 6$) of colonic tissue levels. IBD significantly ($P < 0.05$, $n = 6$) decreased mean colonic tissue levels of GSH to 22.34 ± 3.20 μM on day 4 of IBD. There was a non-significant reduction in mean colonic tissue levels of GSH on days 2 and 7 of IBD. Administration of NRD 30 minutes after the induction of IBD, significantly ($P < 0.05$, $P < 0.01$) increased mean GSH colonic levels on days 4 and 7, respectively. After 2 days of IBD, there was a non-significant increase in mean colonic tissue levels of GSH. There was a significant ($P < 0.05$, $n = 6$) increase in mean colonic tissue levels of GSH, after

oral administration of NRD for 3 days before the induction of IBD. There was an increase in mean colonic tissue levels of GSH on day 4 but increased non-significantly after 2 and 7 days of IBD.

Effect of nerolidol on catalase activity in acetic acid-induced IBD

In order to examine the protective effect of NRD against oxidative stress, we measured colonic catalase (CAT) tissue levels after the administration of NRD either 3 days before or 30 min after the induction of IBD in rats (Fig. 4b). Catalase is an antioxidative enzyme located in peroxisomes that safely decomposes superoxide anions and thus protects against oxidative stress. Before the induction of IBD, colonic tissue catalase activity level in the untreated control group (no IBD, no NRD) was 2.13 ± 0.20 nmol/min/mg protein. There was a significant ($P < 0.001$, no NRD, $n = 6$) increase in mean colonic tissue catalase activity after the induction of IBD on all the days tested. NRD had a non-significant ($P > 0.05$) effect on catalase colonic tissue activity, when administered orally 30 min after the induction of IBD, on all the days tested. However, administration of NRD 3 days before the induction of IBD, significantly ($P < 0.001$, $n = 6$) increased the catalase colonic tissue activity only on day 7, from 6.60 ± 0.31 (no NRD) to 10.24 ± 0.48 nmol/min/mg of protein. NRD had no effect on colonic catalase tissue activity on days 4 and 7 of IBD.

Effect of nerolidol on mean superoxide dismutase activity in acetic acid-induced IBD

Superoxide dismutase (SOD), a metal ion cofactor-requiring enzyme, is an antioxidant enzyme that protects against oxidative stress. To test whether NRD has any effect on SOD, it was administered either 3 days pre- or 30 min post-IBD in rats (Fig. 4c). There was a significant ($P < 0.05$, IBD, no NRD, $n=6$) increase in mean colonic superoxide dismutase activity 4 days post-IBD. The activity level of superoxide dismutase was unaffected on days 2 and 7 of IBD. Administration of NRD after the induction of IBD, significantly ($P < 0.05$), $n = 6$ increased mean colonic SOD activity level on days 2 and 7 of IBD, respectively. The activity level of SOD was unaffected by NRD on day 4 of IBD. There was a significant ($P < 0.05$, $n = 6$) increase in SOD activity level when NRD was administered before IBD. Pre-treated NRD had no effect on the superoxide dismutase activity on day 4 of IBD.

Effect of nerolidol on mean malondialdehyde levels in acetic acid-induced IBD

Malondialdehyde (MDA), a highly reactive compound generated by peroxidation of membrane polyunsaturated fatty acids, is a marker for oxidative stress. In order to measure the effects of NRD on mean MDA levels in the colonic tissues, it was administered either 3 days pre- or 30 min post-IBD and continued for 7 days in rats (Fig. 4d). There was a significant ($P < 0.001$, $n=6$) increase in mean colonic tissue levels of MDA after the IBD induction, on day 2. IBD had no effect on the MDA levels on days 4 and 7. Post-IBD administration of NRD significantly ($P < 0.01$, $n = 6$) deceased MDA levels on day 2 of IBD. The mean colonic tissue levels of MDA were unaffected by NRD after 4 and 7 days of IBD. Administration of NRD 3 days before IBD, significantly ($P < 0.001$, $n = 6$) decreased MDA levels on day 2 but had no effect on MDA levels on days 4 and 7 of IBD.

a

b

Fig. 2 (a) Light micrographs of the colon of rats showing the effects of nerolidol on IBD-induced lesions. **A**: Naïve (control); (**B**) 1: 2-day IBD control—no nerolidol, 2: 2-day IBD, post-treated with nerolidol, 3: 2-day IBD (pretreated). (**C**) 1: 4-day IBD control – no nerolidol, 2: 4-day IBD, post-treated with nerolidol 3: 4-day IBD (pretreated). (**D**) 1: 7-day IBD control – no nerolidol, 2: 7-day IBD, post-treated with nerolidol, 3: 7-day IBD (pretreated). (**b**) Effect of nerolidol on microscopic Ulcer score in IBD rat model. Data are presented as mean ± SEM. *Significant difference between nerolidol-treated and non-IBD control. #Significant difference between nerolidol-treated and IBD control. * $P< 0.05$, ***$P < 0.001$ vs. non-IBD control group; #$P < 0.05$, ##$P < 0.01$ vs. relative IBD control group

Effect of nerolidol on interleukin-1 (IL-1β) levels in acetic acid-induced IBD

Interleukin-1 (IL-1β), also known as leukocyte pyrogen or leukocyte endogenous factor, is a cytokine protein and a mediator of colonic inflammation. To examine whether the administration of NRD has any effects on colonic tissue levels of interleukin-1 (IL-1β), after it was administered either pre- or post-IBD in rats (Fig. 5a). There was a significant ($P < 0.05$, $P < 0.001$, $n=6$) increase in colonic tissue levels of IL-1β levels after IBD after 2 and 4 days of IBD, respectively. Mean colonic tissue IL-1β levels were unaffected by NRD on day 7 of IBD. However, post-IBD administration of NRD resulted in a significant ($P < 0.05$, $P < 0.001$, $n = 6$) reduction in mean colonic tissue levels of IL-1β levels 2 and 4 days after the induction of IBD, respectively. After 7 days of IBD, colonic tissue levels of IL-1β were seen unaffected by administration of NRD. Pre-IBD administration of NRD significantly ($P < 0.05$, $P < 0.001$, $n = 6$) reduced the colonic tissue levels of IL-1β in untreated group (IBD, no NRD), as well as 2 and 4 days after the induction of IBD, respectively. Pre-IBD administration of NRD had no effect on colonic tissue levels of IL-1β after 7 days of IBD.

Effect of nerolidol on interleukin-23 levels in acetic acid-induced IBD

Interleukin-23 (IL-23) is the key mediator of intestinal inflammation. To determine whether NRD has any effect on mean colonic tissue levels of IL-23, NRD was administered either 3 days before or 30 min after the induction of IBD (Fig. 5b). In the control group (no IBD, no NRD), IL-23 level was 14.19 ± 2.21 pg/mg of protein. After 2 days of IBD induction, there was a non-significant increase in IL-23 colonic tissue levels on day 2 but a significant increase ($P < 0.05$, $P < 0.01$) after 4 and 7 days of IBD (control, No NRD). Administration of NRD after the induction of IBD had a significant ($P < 0.05$, $n = 6$) effect on colonic tissue levels of IL-23 only after 4 days but no effect on days 2

and 7 of IBD. There was a significantly ($P < 0.05$, $P < 0.01$, $n = 6$) reduction in the colonic tissue levels of IL-23 when NRD was administered pre-IBD on days 4 and 7. NRD had no effect on mean colonic IL-23 tissue levels on day 2 of IBD.

Effect of nerolidol on interleukin-6 levels in acetic acid-induced IBD

Interleukin-6 (IL-6), is a pro-inflammatory cytokine in the intestine but anti-inflammatory myokine in skeletal muscles. In order to study the effect of NRD on IL-6, it was administered either 3 days pre- or 30 min post-IBD (Fig. 5c). Mean colonic tissue levels of IL-6 was significantly ($P < 0.01$, $P < 0.001$, $n = 6$) increased by IBD. Moreover, there was a significant ($P < 0.05$, $P < 0.001$, $n = 6$) increase in mean colonic tissue levels of IL-6 when NRD was administered post-IBD. Administration of NRD 3 days pre-IBD, significantly ($P < 0.05$, $P < 0.01$, $n = 6$) increased the mean colonic tissue levels of IL-6 in the untreated group (IBD, no NRD), as well as after 2 and 4 days of IBD, respectively. Colonic tissue levels of IL-6 on day 7 was unaffected by NRD administered 3 days before IBD.

Effect of nerolidol on mean TNF-α levels in acetic acid-induced IBD

Tumor necrosis factor-α (TNF-α) is a cell signaling protein involved in systemic inflammation and is one of the cytokines that make up the acute phase reaction. To measure its involvement in AA-induced inflammation, NRD was administered either 3 days pre- or 30 min post-IBD in rats (Fig. 5d). There was a significant ($P < 0.05$, $n=6$) decrease in mean colonic levels of TNF-α (IBD, no NRD) on day of IBD. It decreased only on day 4. IBD had no effect on mean colonic TNF-α levels after days 2 and 7. Mean colonic levels of TNF-α were unaffected by the administration of NRD either pre- or post-IBD, on all the days tested.

Fig. 3 Effect of nerolidol on calprotectin levels in colon. Data are presented as mean ± SEM. *Significant difference between nerolidol-treated and non-IBD control. #Significant difference between nerolidol-treated and IBD control. *$P < 0.05$, ***$P < 0.001$; ##$P < 0.01$, ###$P < 0.001$

Fig. 4 Effect of nerolidol on a GSH, b catalase, c SOD and d MDA in colon. Data are presented as mean ± SEM. *Significant difference between nerolidol-treated and non-IBD control. #Significant difference between nerolidol-treated and IBD control. *$P < 0.05$, **$P < 0.01$, *** $P < 0.001$; #$P < 0.05$, ##$P < 0.01$, ###$P < 0.001$

Fig. 5 Effect of nerolidol on pro-inflammatory cytokines a IL-1β, b IL-23, c Il-6 and d TNF-α in colon. Data are presented as mean ± SEM. *Significant difference between nerolidol-treated and non-IBD control. # Significant difference between nerolidol-treated and IBD control. *$P < 0.05$, **$P < 0.01$ ***$P < 0.001$; #$P < 0.05$, ##$P < 0.01$, ###$P < 0.001$

Table 2　Effect of nerolidol (NRD) on MPO activity (ng/mg protein) in IBD rat model

Dose (mg/kg)	Non-IBD control	IBD control	IBD post-nerolidol-treated	Pre-IBD nerolidol-treated
Day 0 Control	24.30 ± 7.72			
Day 2		45686.36 ± 9180.63***	2958 ± 784.93##	3149.64 ± 892.25##
Day 4		462.45 ± 133.86**	159.57 ± 1.46#	191.29 ± 21.56#
Day 7		117.80 ± 30.03***	89.03 ± 15.29	54.05 ± 3.81

***$P < 0.001$ day 0 non IBD control group vs IBD control group; #$P < 0.05$, ##$P < 0.01$, ###$P < 0.001$, IBD control group vs post/pre-treatment

Effect of nerolidol on mean myeloperoxidase (MPO) activity in acetic acid-induced IBD

Myeloperoxidase (MPO) is a heme-enzyme localized in lysosomes of neutrophils, macrophages and monocytes. Increased activity is also found in inflamed mucosa in ulcerative colitis. Therefore, to measure its activity in colonic tissues and the extent of neutrophil migration to the site of inflammation, NRD was administered either 3 days pre- or 30 min post-IBD (Table 2). There was a significant ($P < 0.01$, $P < 0.001$) increase in colonic tissue activity of MPO in control group (IBD, no NRD) on days 2, 4 and 7 of IBD, respectively. However, there was a significant ($P < 0.05$, $P < 0.01$, $n = 6$) reduction in colonic tissue activity of MPO when NRD was administered post-IBD. NRD had no effect on mean colonic tissue activity of MPO on day 7 of IBD. Moreover, mean colonic tissue activity of MPO was significantly ($P < 0.05$, $P < 0.01$, $n = 6$) reduced when NRD was administered 3 days Pre-IBD. Mean colonic tissue activity of MPO was unaffected by NRD on day 7 of IBD.

DISCUSSION

The result of our study shows that NRD effectively improved body weight, colonic length by attenuating oxidative stress, and inflammation. Furthermore, the preservation and protection of colonic mucosa by NRD clearly show its usefulness in AA-induced colitis in rats.

Recent insights into the role of oxidative stress in IBD have shed light in improving therapy in IBD, particularly the health benefits of plants as well as plant-derived phytochemicals due to their antioxidant and anti-inflammatory properties. These natural antioxidants are believed to impede the progression of disease, as well as rescue patients from the disease. The results of the present findings also suggest that NRD could be a useful agent in the treatment of IBD. This is the first report to demonstrate the protective eff of NRD on acetic acid-induced in rats in line with various other terpene compounds such as geraniol, carvacrol, menthol, betulinic acid, celastrol, and eucalyptol by suppressing inflammatory process in animal models of IBD.

The rat model of AA-induced colitis used in the present study is a widely used animal model for testing the effectiveness of different agents that target inflammation and oxidative stress. This model mimics the pathogenesis of clinical IBD. The result of the present study showed that IBD altered the epithelial integrity and colonic injury by modulating the mucosal immune system following neutrophil and macrophage infiltrations. Despite the mucoprotective barrier of the epithelial layer, ingested materials or pathogens activate the mucosal epithelium, polymorphonuclear neutrophils, and macrophages to produce pro-inflammatory cytokines and other mediators that affect colon mucosa integrity. In the present study, induction of IBD by 4% AA caused a high degree of inflammation, loss of goblet cell, and colon tissue injury due to infiltration of the surface epithelium by leucocytes, which is well supported by the histopathology observations. The reduction in body weight and changes in the length of the colon tissue in rats are sensitive indicators of the extent and severity of inflammatory responses. In the present study, improved body weight, colon length, and reduced diarrhea following treatment with NRD illustrate its usefulness in ulcerative colitis and the possibility of other terpene compounds for possible use as therapeutic agents in colitis.

Treatment with NRD attenuated the macroscopic and microscopic injury in the colonic tissue of rat as observed histologically. The preservation of epithelial goblet cells, which produce mucin, is the main reason for reduced tissue damage. Vascular mechanisms and mucin, a glucoprotein, play an important role in the protection and healing of gut mucosa. Studies have shown that low mucosal blood flow predisposes to injury, whereas increase in blood flow protects against noxious agents. The mechanism of protection involves supply of oxygen and bicarbonate (HCO^-_3) and the prevention of deleterious agents entering the mucosa. Alteration in the balance between the production of ROS and detoxification by endogenous antioxidant defense system are factors that lead to intestinal damage in IBD. In normal physiological circumstances, the colonic mucosa keeps the level of endogenous antioxidant enzymes activity balanced in such a precise manner that it is enough to keep the levels of ROS low. In situation where there is an increased level of ROS (H_2O_2) due to decrease in its removal, an alternative reaction occurs which results in increased levels of cellular hydroxyl radical ($OH^•$) or hypochlorous acid (HOCl) which lead to impaired epithelial cell integrity, impeding mucosal recovery, and increasing intestinal mucosal permeability. This results in reduced barrier function and host defense leading to the infiltration of bacteria and microorganisms, which in turn releases a large amount of reactive oxygen metabolites. Endogenous antioxidant enzymes such as SOD and CAT and a non-enzymatic antioxidant, GSH, protect cells and organisms from cytotoxic reactive oxygen and reactive nitrogen species. SODs are metal ion cofactor-requiring enzymes that catalyzes the dismutation of $O2^{•-}$ into O_2 and H_2O_2. The uncharged H_2O_2 in the cytosol is further converted into water by CAT, a heme-enzyme located in peroxisomes, or enzymes of the glutathione redox cycle, a component of endogenous antioxidant defense system.

The present study showed that NRD, by increasing the tissue levels of SOD and CAT, prevented excessive free radical generation and reduced the formation of lipid peroxides and aldehyde, MDA, in AA-induced colitis. GSH, a tripeptide with a reactive sulphydryl group, plays an important role in detoxification by inhibiting ROS, facilitating the synthesis and repair of DNA, thus reducing the risk of colon cancer, enhances the promotion of the recycling of endogenous anti-oxidants, and subsequently improves vitamin C antioxidant activity and enhances amino acids transport. Despite being a substrate for antioxidant enzyme, GPx, GSH scavenges several reactive oxygen metabolites including $O2^{•-}$, $OH^•$, peroxynitrite, and hydroperoxides. During its function as an antioxidant, reduced GSH is converted to its oxidized state. Subsequently, it is reduced back to GSH by glutathione reductase. A reduced level of GSH in colonic tissues indicates occurrence of oxidative stress and enhanced level of GSH following treatment with NRD demonstrate its antioxidant properties in colitis. NRD has been shown to interfere with ROS production and restore the levels of GSH bioavailability leading to a reduction of ethanol- and indomethacin-induced mucosal damage, stress-induced gastric ulcer, as well as in heart, brain and lungs.

In addition to reduced antioxidant defense, there was an increased formation of lipid peroxides following lipid peroxidation of membranes which was characterized by increased colonic tissue levels of malondialdehyde (MDA) in AA-challenged animals. This explains its usage as an indicator of oxidative stress in cells and tissues besides myeloperoxidase (MPO). MDA is a naturally occurring product of lipid peroxidation; it can also be generated during prostaglandin biosynthesis in cells. An increase in free radical causes overproduction of MDA. Lipid peroxidation is a process under which oxidants such as free radicals inflict direct damage on membrane lipids containing carbon–carbon double bonds, especially polyunsaturated fatty acids (PUFAs). It also affects other lipids, proteins, and DNA. ROS initiates lipid peroxidation by removing a hydrogen atom. Previous studies have shown that MDA levels are elevated in IBD peroxidation. Furthermore, there has been an increased report of lipid peroxidation in AA-induced tissue injuries, which is similar to the findings of the present study. Therefore, substances which prevent the formation ROS or potentiate the endogenous enzymatic or non-enzymatic anti-oxidant systems can have beneficial effects in reducing intestinal inflammation and damage in ulcerative colitis. Similarly, NRD has been shown to enhance antioxidant enzymes, inhibit lipid peroxidation, and bring a reduction in the infiltration of inflammatory cells (neutrophils) in various other tissues.

Under normal conditions, there is a tight-control in the balance between pro-inflammatory (IL-1β, IL-6, IL-8, IL-17, IL-23, and TNF-α) and anti-inflammatory (IL-5, IL-10, IL-11, and TGF-β) cytokines in the mucosa of the gastrointestinal (GI) tract. The secretion of pro-inflammatory cytokines is initiated by macrophages and neutrophils, which activate the adaptive immune system. This results in the disruption of the balance between T-helper (Th) cells and intolerant regulatory T cells, leading to initiation and progression of inflammation in colonic tissues. Crohn's disease is characterized by Th1 cell-mediated inflammation of the colonic mucosa with increased level of IL-12, IL-17, and IL-23 cytokines while ulcerative colitis is influenced by IL-4, IL-5, IL-10, and IL-13 produced by Th2- type T cells. Increased colonic tissue level of IL-1β, IL-23, and TNF-α is often used as a biomarker for the severity of colitis. IL-1β is made mainly by monocytes, tissue macrophages, and various other cells, are involved in myriad immunological responses spanning both innate and adaptive immunity. IL-1β production, which is synthetized in inactive form and activated by caspase-1, is initiated by cyclooxygenase type 2, phospholipase A, and iNOS. In contrast to other cytokines, IL-6 is a pleiotropic cytokine that acts both as pro-inflammatory cytokine and an anti-inflammatory myokine. Recent evidence has suggested that IL-6 may play an important role in driving chronic inflammation, autoimmunity, endothelial dysfunction by activated macrophages, and colon epithelial cells to secrete inflammatory cytokines. TNF-α, released mainly from activated macrophages, disrupts intestinal epithelial barrier, induces apoptosis of epithelial cells, promotes ROS production, activates neutrophils, and plays an important role in the pathogenesis of IBD. TNF-α is a critical cytokine that facilitates the generation of superoxides in colon epithelial cells by activating NOX1 and NADPH oxidase organizer 1 (NOXO1). Activation of NOX1, and ROs generation are all involved in activating NF-kB by TNF-α. Activation of NOX1, ROs generation, and IkBa are all involved in activating NF-kB through TNF-α. Research has shown that oxidative stress is involved in activation of NF-κB signaling in IBD which can elevate the transcription of different types of genes that are instrumental in the pathogenesis of IBD.

NRD has been shown to have anti-inflammatory effects by downregulating the expression of inflammatory mediators and signaling pathways such as inhibition of LOX-1/IL-1β and TLR4/NF-κB signaling and AMPK/ Nrf-2/ HO-1 pathway. The anti-inflammatory activities observed in the present study are in line with previous reports wherein NRD showed potent anti-inflammatory activity by inhibiting the release and secretion of proinflammatory cytokines in brain, kidney, liver, heart, lungs, testes, uterus, stomach, and ocular tissues. Based on the results of the present study and studies conducted by other workers, NRD is found to be beneficial in IBD and like other herbal anti-inflammatory agents, NRD does not cause gastrointestinal adverse effects and appears safer than conventional anti-inflammatory drugs.

Polymorphonuclear infiltration of the colonic tissue was reduced when the rats were treated with NRD, which was evidenced by microscopic examination and significant reduction in MPO activity. NRD appears to inhibit leukocyte and neutrophil migration and, in addition, inhibits the rolling and adhesion of leukocytes in colon tissues. Neutrophil and macrophage infiltrate into AA-induced damaged sites in colon tissues and the degree of tissue infiltration depends on the activity of MPO. This enzyme is mainly found in primary granules of neutrophils in humans and to a lesser extent in monocytes and macrophages. The degree of MPO activity serves as the bases for quantitative assay for acute inflammation of the intestine, which is a measure of neutrophil infiltration. The primary granules of neutrophils release MPO, a heme-containing enzyme, during inflammation which catalyzes H_2O_2-dependent peroxidation of Cl^-, HOCl, which exert antimicrobial properties. The reactive oxygen species formed in this process are responsible for intracellular damages to host cells targeting carbohydrates, proteins, nucleic acids, and lipids. Neutrophils and macrophages exhibit prominent roles during mucosal inflammation by producing superoxide and nitric oxide (NO) by activating NOX and iNOS, respectively, leading to barrier dysfunction and tissue necrosis.

Furthermore, in this study, decreased calprotectin following NRD treatment demonstrated the protective effects of NRD on colonic tissues. Calprotectin is associated with inflammation and is derived from neutrophils and studies have shown an increased tissue levels of calprotectin in patients with IBD and fetal calprotectin accurately predicts relapse. Wide margin of safety and negligible adverse effects of NRD indicates its safety and the beneficial effect following oral route of administration further indicates its convenient dosage form for therapeutic and nutritional use in humans.

There is a clear evidence for the protective role of NRD on AA-induced colitis in rats by macroscopic and biochemical observations, which is well supported by the histopathological studies. In the present study, AA, administered rectally, resulted in severe inflammation and necrosis of the colonic mucosa, reduced colonic length, increased inflammatory cell infiltration with edema, and caused occasional hyperemia and goblet cell hyperplasia as observed in the histopathological studies. These observations, which characterize IBD, are consistent with our studies done previously using similar animal model. NRD treatment remarkably improved the colonic histoarchitecture by preserving microscopic and macroscopic structures of colon and preventing depletion of colonic wall mucosa. Pretreatment with NRD resulted in reduction of the histological signs of inflammation, namely leukocyte infiltration, edema, and tissue injury. The observation of the present study wherein NRD protects against AA-induced colitis is in support of other studies done with ethanol, NSAIDs such as indomethacin, and stress-induced gastric lesion where the mean gastric lesion area was significantly reduced.

Integrating the anticancer activity in cancer cells of the colon by suppressing cell growth, cell proliferation, and induction of apoptosis without affecting the integrity of normal cells as well as antiulcer, antioxidant, and anti-inflammatory potential, NRD appears to be a promising molecule for its therapeutic potential in colitis, a risk factor of colon cancer. Additionally, the results of our study also provide scientific validation of traditional claims of plants containing NRD for the treatment of diseases of the gastrointestinal tract.

This study reveals the potent antioxidant and anti-inflammatory effects of NRD in an acute colon inflammation model induced by AA. Considering the safety of NRD and demonstrated efficacy of NRD in gastric as well as colon tissues, the results of the present study provide a foundation for further investigations on molecular mechanism and it can be a promising phytochemical agent for nutraceutical or development of pharmaceuticals in IBD.

JOURNAL ARTICLE EXERCISE 2

Remember that the science sections on the MCAT include a significant number of passages with experiments. You'll need to be able to extract information efficiently and analyze data effectively in order to do well on these passages.

This is the second of three "Journal Article Exercises" in this book. In the first exercise, we showed you the type of information you should be able to extract from the article and the sorts of things to pay attention to in the data. In this exercise, you'll do more of that on your own, and in the final exercise we'll show you how that article might get turned into an MCAT-style passage.

As a reminder, when analyzing an experiment, you should be able to:

- identify the control group(s).
- extract information from graphs and data tables.
- determine how the experimental group(s) change relative to the control.
- determine if the results are statistically significant.
- come to a reasonable conclusion about WHY the results were observed.
- consider potential weaknesses in the study.
- determine how to increase the power of the study.
- decide what the next most logical experiment or study should be.

Again, the goal of these exercises is NOT to learn content from the articles, just to get a little more comfortable reading and extracting information from them.

For the (abridged) article on pages 171–181, try to summarize the purpose of the experiment and the methods in 4–5 sentences. Consider the following mnemonic: Oh ouR Car Won't Start (ORCWS).

- **O = Organism and Organization**: is the research being conducted on humans or on animals or on bacteria, or something else? What is being done to these organisms? Are there any unique qualities to these organisms? Are there multiple groups? Is the study conducted over a long period of time with multiple data points, or is it a short-term study? Does it have a large or small n?
- **R = Results**: where and how are the results presented? Is it a graph? A data table? Figures and images? What is/are the independent variable(s)? What is/are the dependent variable(s)? Do the results show correlation or cause and effect, or both? Describe.
- **C = Control and Comparison**: is there a control group? How does it differ from the experimental group? Is it given a placebo or nothing at all? Is it held under different conditions? If there are multiple experimental groups, how do they differ from one another? Is it a blinded study? If so, double-blind or single-blind?
- **W = Weirdness**: does anything or do any of the results stand out as unexpected?
- **S = Statistics**: was any sort of statistical analysis done? How is it presented? Are there error bars on a graph? Standard errors around a mean? Are there p-values? Is there an asterisk indicating statistical significance? Is there any data that is not statistically significant?

Try interpreting the data on your own before reading the results/discussion section. When you do read the discussion, consider:

- What are the conclusions of the study?
- How are the conclusions supported by the data?
- What potential weaknesses or flaws do you see in the experimental design? Are these addressed in the discussion section?
- How might this study be potentially biased?
- How might this study be improved?
- What would be the next most logical experiment?

Answer these questions for the article on pages 171–181.

1. **O = Organism and Organization:**
    - Is the research being conducted on humans or on animals or on bacteria in a petri dish, or something else?
      _____
      _____

    - What is being done to these organisms?
      _____
      _____

    - Are there any unique qualities to these organisms?
      _____
      _____

    - Are there multiple groups?
      _____
      _____

    - Is the study conducted over a long period of time with multiple data points, or is it a short-term study?
      _____
      _____

    - Does it have a large or small n?
      _____
      _____

2. **R = Results:**
    - Where and how are the results presented? Is it a graph? A data table? Figures and images?
      _____
      _____

    - What is/are the independent variable(s)?
      _____
      _____

    - What is/are the dependent variable(s)?
      _____
      _____

    - What are the results of the study?
      _____
      _____

     • Do the results show correlation or cause and effect, or both? Describe.

_____

_____

3. **C = Control and Comparison:**
   • Is there a control group?

_____

_____

   • How does it differ from the experimental group? Is it given a placebo or nothing at all? Is it held under different conditions?

_____

_____

   • If there are multiple experimental groups, how do they differ from one another?

_____

_____

   • Is it a blinded study? If so, double blind or single blind?

_____

_____

4. **W = Weirdness:**
   • Does anything or do any of the results stand out as unexpected?

_____

_____

5. **S = Statistics:**
   • Was any sort of statistical analysis done?

_____

_____

   • How is it presented? Are there error bars on a graph? Standard errors around a mean? Are there p-values? Is there an asterisk indicating statistical significance?

_____

_____

   • Is there any data that is not statistically significant?

_____

_____

6. **Interpreting the data:**
   • What are the conclusions of the study?

_____

_____

- How are the conclusions supported by the data?

  _____

  _____

- What potential weaknesses or flaws do you see in the experimental design? Are these addressed in the discussion section?

  _____

  _____

- How might this study be potentially biased?

  _____

  _____

- How might this study be improved?

  _____

  _____

- What would be the next most logical experiment?

  _____

  _____

7. **Final Summary of Experiment and Results:**

   _____

   _____

   _____

   _____

   _____

   _____

SOLUTIONS TO JOURNAL ARTICLE EXERCISE 2

1. **O = Organism and Organization:**
   - Is the research being conducted on humans or on animals or on bacteria in a petri dish, or something else? *Rats.*
   - What is being done to these organisms? *Colitis is induced and the effect of nerolidol (a terpene found in tea) is assessed (both as a treatment and as a preventative).*
   - Are there any unique qualities to these organisms? *No.*
   - Are there multiple groups? *Yes. Control, pre-colitis treatment, and post-colitis treatment*
   - Is the study conducted over a long period of time with multiple data points, or is it a short-term study? *Short term (7–10 days), several data points within those 7–10 days*
   - Does it have a large or small *n*? *small n: 18 animals per group.*

2. **R = Results:**
   - Where and how are the results presented? Is it a graph? A data table? Figures and images? *Photos and graphs*
   - What is/are the independent variable(s)? *Nerolidol*
   - What is/are the dependent variable(s)? *Ulceration (severity of colitis), body weight, calprotectin levels, glutathione levels, catalase activity, superoxide dismutase activity, malondialdehyde levels, interleukin levels, tumor necrosis factor levels, myeloperoxidase activity.*
   - What are the results of the study? *The rats treated with nerolidol, both after induction of colitis and as a pretreatment, showed less tissue damage, less oxidative damage, and lower levels of inflammatory markers.*
   - Do the results show correlation or cause and effect, or both? Describe. *Cause and effect: treatment of rats with nerolidol reduced the effects of the induced colitis.*

3. **C = Control and Comparison:**
   - Is there a control group? *Yes*
   - How does it differ from the experimental group? Is it given a placebo or nothing at all? Is it held under different conditions? *There were two control groups: one that was not induced to colitis and one that was induced to colitis and not treated with nerolidol.*
   - If there are multiple experimental groups, how do they differ from one another? *There were two experimental groups, one that was pretreated with nerolidol before induction of colitis and one that was treated with nerolidol after induction of colitis.*
   - Is it a blinded study? If so, double blind or single blind? *Not a blinded study*

4. **W = Weirdness:**
   - Does anything or do any of the results stand out as unexpected? *Not all inflammatory cytokine levels are reduced. Il-6 was increased in nerolidol treated rats.*

5. **S = Statistics:**
   - Was any sort of statistical analysis done? *Yes*
   - How is it presented? Are there error bars on a graph? Standard errors around a mean? Are there *p*-values? Is there an asterisk indicating statistical significance? *P values, error bars, asterisks*
   - Is there any data that is not statistically significant? *There are a few measures that are not statistically significant, e.g., IL-23 levels 2 days after induction of colitis. TNF-α levels are generally not statistically significant.*

6. **Interpreting the data:**
   - What are the conclusions of the study? *Generally speaking, treatment with nerolidol reduces tissue damage and levels of inflammatory markers, while increasing levels of anti-oxidant enzymes.*
   - How are the conclusions supported by the data? *Data on tissue damage and levels of inflammatory markers and antioxidant enzymes show significant differences between treated and untreated groups.*
   - What potential weaknesses or flaws do you see in the experimental design? Are these addressed in the discussion section? *Treatment was on animals; results do not always transfer to humans.*
   - How might this study be potentially biased? *These studies were done previously with similar animal models; the researchers may have been biased in looking for/expecting positive results.*
   - How might this study be improved? *No obvious ways to improve the study.*
   - What would be the next most logical experiment? *Repeat the experiment, but compare treatment with nerolidol to treatment with other anti-inflammatory agents. Study the effects of nerolidol treatment in humans with IBD or ulcerative colitis.*

7. **Final Summary of Experiment and Results:**
   - *In this study, colitis was induced in rats by the application of acetic acid. Some rats were treated prophylactically with nerolidol prior to induction of colitis, and some rats were treated with nerolidol after induction of colitis. In all cases, tissue damage and inflammation were reduced by nerolidol. No adverse effects of nerolidol treatment occurred. This points to nerolidol, a plant compound, as a reasonable treatment for IBD and colitis in humans.*

Chapter 7
Nucleic Acids

The biological macromolecules are grouped into four classes of molecules that play important roles in cells and in organisms as a whole. All of them are polymers—strings of repeated units (monomers).

This chapter discusses the nucleic acids from a biological perspective: what they are made of, how they are put together, and what their roles are in the body. These molecules are also discussed in *MCAT Organic Chemistry Review* from an organic chemistry perspective: nomenclature, chirality, etc.

7.1 PHOSPHORUS-CONTAINING COMPOUNDS

Phosphoric acid is an *inorganic* acid (it does not contain carbon) with the potential to donate three protons. The pK_as for the three acid dissociation equilibria are 2.1, 7.2, and 12.4. Therefore, at physiological pH, phosphoric acid is significantly dissociated, existing largely in anionic form. The most common species (approximately 60% in extracellular fluid) is hydrogen phosphate (HPO_4^{-2}), and the second most common (approximately 40%) is dihydrogen phosphate ($H_2PO_4^{-}$).

Figure 1 Phosphoric Acid Dissociation

Phosphate is also known as orthophosphate. Two orthophosphates bound together via an **anhydride linkage** form **pyrophosphate**. The P–O–P bond in pyrophosphate is an example of a **high-energy phosphate bond**. This name is derived from the fact that the hydrolysis of pyrophosphate is thermodynamically extremely favorable. The $\Delta G°$ for the hydrolysis of pyrophosphate is about –7 kcal/mol. This means that it is a very favorable reaction. The actual ΔG in the cell is about –12 kcal/mol, which is even more favorable. How is this possible?[1]

There are three reasons that phosphate anhydride bonds store so much energy:

1) When phosphates are linked together, their negative charges repel each other strongly.
2) Orthophosphate has more resonance forms and thus a lower free energy than linked phosphates.
3) Orthophosphate has a more favorable interaction with the biological solvent (water) than linked phosphates.

The details are not crucial. What is essential is that you fix the image in your mind of linked phosphates acting like compressed springs, just waiting to fly open and provide energy for an enzyme to catalyze a reaction.

Figure 2 The Hydrolysis of Pyrophosphate

---

[1] Remember from Chapter 3 that $\Delta G°$ is the free energy change at standard conditions. The concentrations of reactants and products inside the cell are not at standard conditions. In fact, the cell maintains a concentration of ATP much higher than that of ADP and phosphate, which makes ATP hydrolysis so much more favorable.

Nucleotides

Nucleotides are the building blocks of nucleic acids (RNA and DNA). Each nucleotide contains a **ribose** (or **deoxyribose**) **sugar** group; a **purine** or **pyrimidine base** joined to carbon number one of the ribose ring; and one, two, or three phosphate units joined to carbon five of the ribose ring. The nucleotide **a**denosine **tri**phosphate (ATP) plays a central role in cellular metabolism in addition to being an RNA precursor. Significantly more information about the function of the nucleic acids RNA and DNA will be provided in *MCAT Biology Review*.

ATP is the universal short-term energy storage molecule. It is a ribonucleotide (ribose is the sugar, as opposed to deoxyribose). Energy extracted from the oxidation of foodstuffs is immediately stored in the phospho-anhydride bonds of ATP. This energy is used to power cellular processes, and as we have already seen, it may also be used to synthesize glucose or fats, which are longer-term energy storage molecules. This applies to *all* living organisms, from bacteria to humans. Even some viruses carry ATP with them outside the host cell, though viruses cannot make their own ATP.

Figure 3   Adenosine Triphosphate (ATP)

The other nucleotides can also be used as energy (high-energy phosphate is high-energy phosphate, after all!), but they are used for this purpose far less often. GTP is used for energy in protein synthesis, and UTP is used to activate glucose-1-P in glycogenesis.

7.2 DNA STRUCTURE

General Overview

Understanding the structure of DNA provides great insight into its function, so let's start at the smallest level and work our way up. DNA is short for deoxyribonucleic acid. DNA and RNA (ribonucleic acid) are called **nucleic acids** because they are found in the nucleus and possess many acidic phosphate groups.

The building block of DNA is the deoxyribonucleoside 5′ triphosphate (dNTP, where N represents one of the four basic nucleosides). Deoxyadenosine 5′ triphosphate (dATP) is shown in Figure 4. Deoxyribonucleotides are built from three components. The first is a simple monosaccharide, deoxyribose. [How does the structure of deoxyribose compare with that of ribose?[2]] In a dNTP, carbons on the ribose are referred to as 1′, 2′, and so on. The next component of the dNTP is an aromatic, nitrogenous base, namely **adenine** (A), **guanine** (G), **cytosine** (C), or **thymine** (T); see Figure 5. (Don't mix up the DNA base thymine with vitamin B₁, thiamine.) These aromatic molecules are bases because they contain several nitrogens which have free electron pairs capable of accepting protons. G and A are derived from a precursor called purine, so they are referred to as the **purines** and have a double-ring structure (a six-membered ring and a five-membered ring). C and T are the **pyrimidines**; they have single six-membered ring structure.[3]

A **nucleo*side*** is ribose (a deoxynucleoside is deoxyribose) with a purine or pyrimidine linked to the 1′ carbon in a β-N-glycosidic linkage. [In the β-N-glycosidic linkage of a nucleoside, is the aromatic base above or is it below the plane of ribose in a Haworth projection?[4]] The nucleosides are named as follows: A-ribose = adenosine, G-ribose = guanosine, C-ribose = cytidine, T-ribose = thymidine, and U-ribose = uridine. Both purines and pyrimidines have abundant hydrogen bonding potential. [Will adenine and thymine H-bond with each other in dilute aqueous solution (0.1 *M*, for example)?[5]]

The final component of the deoxyribonucleotide building block of DNA is a phosphate group. **Nucleo*tides*** are phosphate esters of nucleosides, with one, two, or three phosphate groups joined to the ribose ring by the 5′ hydroxy group. When nucleotides contain three phosphate residues, they may also be referred to as **deoxynucleoside triphosphates**; they are abbreviated **dNTP**, where d is for *deoxy* and N is for *nucleoside*. In individual nucleotides, N is replaced by A, G, C, T, or U. Because they contain acidic phosphates, the nucleotides may also be referred to by a name ending in "ylate." For example, TTP is thymidylate. The ubiquitous energy molecule, ATP, is a nucleotide which may be called adenylate (it's not deoxy).

---

[2] The 2′ OH is missing in deoxyribose.

[3] A mnemonic for this is: Pyramids (pyrimidines) have sharp edges, so they CUT. The U stands for *uracil*, which is a pyrimidine found in RNA instead of T. Another mnemonic is CUT the Py.

[4] A beta linkage indicates that the anomeric carbon has a configuration with the attached group (a nitrogen of the aromatic ring of a purine or pyrimidine base) drawn *above* the plane of the ribose ring. Remember, it's better to β up!

[5] No. In dilute solution they will be H-bonded to water. However, H-bonds are the key determinant of the double-stranded structure of DNA; in DNA, the bases do not interact with water because DNA coiling places them inside the tube-like structure of the double helix, where they interact with each other.

Figure 4   Deoxyadenosine Triphosphate (dATP)

The sugar-phosphate portion of the nucleotide is referred to as the **backbone** of the nucleic acid because it is invariant. The base is the variable portion of the building block. Thus, there are four different dNTPs, and they differ only in the aromatic base. [What is the backbone in protein, and what is the variable portion of the amino acid?[6] If an enzyme binds to a specific sequence of nucleotides in DNA, will the binding specificity be derived from interactions of portions of the polypeptide enzyme with the ribose and phosphate groups or with the purine and pyrimidine bases?[7]]

---

[6]   Peptide bonds with a carbon between them are the backbone, and the R-group attached to the α carbon is the variable portion.

[7]   Since the backbone is the same regardless of the nucleotide sequence, the specificity in binding must be derived from interactions with bases.

PYRIMIDINE BASES

cytosine

thymine
(DNA only)

uracil
(RNA only)

PURINE BASES

adenine

guanine

Figure 5 Aromatic Bases of DNA and RNA

Polynucleotides

Nucleotides in nucleic acids are covalently linked by **phosphodiester bonds** between the 3′ hydroxy group of the sugar in one nucleotide and the 5′ phosphate group of the sugar in the next nucleotide (Figure 6). [Which reaction is more thermodynamically favorable: the polymerization of nucleoside monophosphates, or the polymerization of nucleoside triphosphates?[8]] A polymer of several nucleotides linked together is termed an *oligo*nucleotide, and a polymer of many nucleotides is a *poly*nucleotide. Since the only unique part of the nucleotide is the base, the sequence of a polynucleotide can be abbreviated by simply listing the bases attached to each nucleotide in the chain. The end of the chain with a free 5′ phosphate group is written first in a polynucleotide, with other nucleotides in the chain indicated in the 5′ to 3′ direction. [Which of the nucleotides in the oligonucleotide ACGT has a free 3′ hydroxy group?[9]]

---

[8] During polymerization of nucleoside triphosphates, pyrophosphate is released and hydrolyzed, driving the polymerization reaction forward. Hydrolysis of the high-energy pyrophosphate molecule makes the polymerization of nucleoside triphosphates more energetically favorable.

[9] The T is written last and is therefore the 3′ nucleotide, or the nucleotide with the free 3′ hydroxy group.

Figure 6   The Polymerization of Nucleotides

The Watson-Crick Model of DNA Structure

James Watson and Francis Crick (with the help of Maurice Wilkins and Rosalind Franklin) developed a model of the structure of DNA in the cell. According to the **Watson-Crick model**, cellular DNA is a right-handed double helix held together by hydrogen bonds and hydrophobic forces between bases. It is important to understand each facet of this model.

In the cell, DNA does not exist in the form of a single long polynucleotide. Instead, the DNA found in the nucleus is double-stranded (**ds**). In ds-DNA, two very long polynucleotide chains are hydrogen-bonded together in an **antiparallel orientation**. Antiparallel means the 5′ end of one chain is paired with the 3′ end of the other. [What common protein structure often depends on H-bonds between antiparallel chains?[10]] The H-bonds in ds-DNA are between the bases on adjacent chains. This H-bonding is very specific: A is always H-bonded to T, and G is always H-bonded to C (Figure 7). Note that this means an H-bonded pair always consists of a *purine plus a pyrimidine*.[11] Thus, both types of base pairs (AT or GC) take up the same amount of room in the DNA double helix. The GC pair is held together by three hydrogen bonds, the AT pair by two. Two chains of DNA are said to be complementary if the bases in each strand can hydrogen bond when the strands are oriented in an antiparallel fashion. If we are talking about ds-DNA 100 nucleotides long, we would say it is 100 base pairs (bp) long. A kbp (kilobase pair) is ds-DNA 1,000 nucleotides long.

Figure 7 Base Pairing

The binding of two complementary strands of DNA into a double-stranded structure is termed **annealing**, or **hybridization**. The separation of strands is termed **melting**, or **denaturation**. The temperature at which a solution of DNA molecules is 50 percent melted is termed the T_m. [Would the T_m of ATTATCAT and its complementary strand be higher than, lower than, or equal to the melting temperature of AGTCGCAT and its complementary strand?[12] If you attached methyl groups to all the acidic phosphate oxygens along the length of a DNA double helix, would the chain have a higher or lower T_m than normal DNA?[13]]

---

[10] Antiparallel H-bonding is reminiscent of the β-pleated sheet, which is a common secondary structure (it can be quaternary, when two separate chains come together to form a sheet).

[11] This fact has a fringe benefit: we can calculate the number of purines if we know the number of pyrimidines. We can actually calculate several variables. Chargoff's rule states that [A] = [T] and [G] = [C]; and [A] + [G] = [T] + [C].

[12] The T_m of the first oligonucleotide pair would be lower because it contains more AT pairs. A and T form only two hydrogen bonds while G and C form three. Thus, it takes less kinetic energy to disrupt A-T rich ds-DNA than G-C rich ds-DNA.

[13] The charged phosphates electrostatically repel each other in normal DNA. Methyl esters will not be charged. The lack of electrostatic repulsion between the methyl ester backbones will increase the T_m, meaning that more kinetic energy will be required to melt the oligonucleotides.

- Which of the following is/are true about ds-DNA?[14]
  - I. If the amount of G in a double helix is known, the amount of C can be calculated.
  - II. If the fraction of purine nucleotides and the total molecular weight of a double helix are known, the amount of cytosine can be calculated.
  - III. The two chains in a piece of ds-DNA containing mostly purines will be bonded together more tightly than the two chains in a piece of ds-DNA containing mostly pyrimidines.
  - IV. The oligonucleotide ATGTAT is complementary to the oligonucleotide ATACAT.

There is another important detail about DNA structure: not only is it double stranded, it is also *coiled*. In ds-DNA, the two hydrogen-bonded antiparallel DNA strands form a **right-handed double helix** (meaning it corkscrews in a clockwise motion) with the bases on the interior and the ribose/phosphate backbone on the exterior. The double helix is stabilized by van der Waals interactions between the bases, which are stacked upon each other. Hydrophobic interactions between the bases are also very important in stabilizing the double helix. [But wait a minute. "Hydro*phobic* interactions between *bases*?" Isn't that a contradiction in terms? How can a *base* be hydro*phobic*?[15]] The bases lie in a plane, perpendicular to the length of the DNA molecule, stacked 3.4 angstroms (Å) apart from each other. The helix pattern repeats itself (i.e., completes a full turn) once every *34 angstroms*, which is every *10 base pairs*. While the length of a DNA double helix may vary enormously, from a few Å in an oligonucleotide to macroscopic lengths in a chromosome, the width is always 20 Å. [If a human chromosome has 9×10^7 base pairs, how long would the chromosome be if it were stretched out completely?[16]]

---

[14] **Item I: True.** For every G, there is a C, and for every A there is a T. Item II: False. The ratio of purines to pyrimidines is always the same (50:50) since each purine is paired with a pyrimidine. In order to calculate the amount of any one base, you have to know the ratio of AT to GC pairs. Item III: False. Again, the ratio of purines to pyrimidines is always the same—50:50. However, two chains containing mostly GC pairs will bond more tightly than two chains containing mostly AT pairs, since GC pairs are held together by 3 H-bonds, while AT pairs have only 2. **Item IV: True.** Remember, the strands are antiparallel: A and T pair, G and C pair, and the 5' end is always written first.

[15] Once a purine is H-bonded to a pyrimidine, most of the polar nature of the individual bases disappears because the charge dipoles are occupied in H-bonds.

[16] Since one angstrom is 10^{-10} meter, the length is $(3.4 \times 10^{-10}$ meters/base pair$)(9 \times 10^7$ base pairs$) = 30 \times 10^{-3}$ meters $= 30$ millimeters.

Figure 8   A Small Section of a DNA Double Helix

Chromosome Structure and Packing

The sum total of an organism's genetic information is called its **genome**. Eukaryotic genomes are composed of several large pieces of linear ds-*DNA*; each piece of ds-DNA is called a **chromosome**. Humans have 46 chromosomes, 23 of which are inherited from each parent. Prokaryotic (bacterial) genomes are composed of a **single circular chromosome**. Viral genomes may be linear or circular DNA or RNA. The human genome consists of over 10^9 base pairs, while bacterial genomes contain only 10^6 base pairs. But there is no direct correlation between genome size and evolutionary sophistication, since the organisms with the largest known genomes are amphibians. Much of the size difference in higher eukaryotic genomes is the result of repetitive DNA that has no known function.

If the DNA remained as a simple double helix floating free in the cell, it would be very bulky and fragile. Prokaryotes have a distinctive mechanism for making their single circular chromosome more compact and sturdy. An enzyme called **DNA gyrase** uses the energy of ATP to twist the gigantic circular molecule. Gyrase functions by breaking the DNA and twisting the two sides of the circle around each other. The resulting structure is a twisted circle that is composed of ds-DNA. As discussed above, the two strands are already coiled, forming a helix. The twists created by DNA gyrase are called **supercoils**, since they are coils of a structure that is already coiled.

Since eukaryotes have even more DNA in their genome than prokaryotes, the eukaryotic genome requires denser packaging to fit within the cell (Figure 9). To accomplish this, eukaryotic DNA is wrapped around globular proteins called **histones**. After being wrapped around histones, but before being completely packed away, DNA has the microscopic appearance of beads on a string. The beads are called **nucleosomes**; they are composed of DNA wrapped around an octamer of histones (a group of eight). The octamer is composed of two units of each of the histone proteins H2A, H2B, H3, and H4. The string between the beads is a length of double-helical DNA called linker DNA and is bound by a single linker histone. Fully packed DNA is called **chromatin**; it is composed of closely stacked nucleosomes. [Based on your knowledge of the interactions of macromolecules and the chemical composition of DNA, do you suppose that histones are mostly basic or mostly acidic?[17]]

Figure 9   DNA Packaging

The following flow summarizes the structure of DNA in the nucleus: **Deoxyribose** → *add base* → **nucleoside** → *add three phosphates* → **nucleotide** → *polymerize with loss of two phosphates* → **oligonucleotide** → *continue polymerization* → **single-stranded polynucleotide** → *two complete chains H-bond in antiparallel orientation* → **ds DNA chain** → *coiling occurs* → **ds helix** → *wrap around histones* → **nucleosomes** → *complete packaging* → **chromatin**.

To look for patterns and morphology, chromosomes can be stained with chemicals. Usually, condensed metaphase chromosomes are used, as they are compact and easier to see. When chromosomes are treated, distinct light and dark regions become visible. The darker regions are denser, and are called **heterochromatin**. Heterochromatin is rich in repeats (see below). The lighter regions are less dense and are called **euchromatin**. Density gives a sense of DNA coiling or compactness, and these patterns are constant and heritable. It's now known that the lighter regions have higher transcription rates and therefore higher gene activity. The looser packing makes DNA accessible to enzymes and proteins.

Giemsa stain can also be used, and it produces what are called "G-banding patterns." Here too, darker staining regions are more dense than lighter staining regions. Chromosome bands are constant and specific to each chromosome, which means they can be used for diagnostic purposes (where cytologists look at chromosome structure). Banding patterns have also been linked to DNA replication, as it's been shown that lighter staining regions start replication earlier than darker staining regions. Again, this is likely due to accessibility of the DNA. Giemsa stains are most often used to produce karyotypes, as shown in Figure 10.

---

[17] They're mostly basic, since they must be attracted to the acidic exterior of the DNA double helix. This basicity is supplied by the amino acids arginine and lysine, which are unusually abundant in histones.

Figure 10   Giemsa Stain (a karyotype)

Centromeres

A centromere is the region of the chromosome to which spindle fibers attach during cell division. The fibers attach via **kinetochores**, multiprotein complexes that act as anchor attachment sites for spindle fibers. Other protein complexes also bind the centromere after DNA replication to keep sister chromatids attached to each other. Centromeres are made of heterochromatin and repetitive DNA sequences. Chromosomes have p (short) and q (long) arms, and the centromere position defines the ratio between the two (Figure 11).

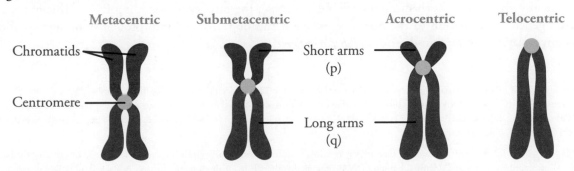

Figure 11   Centromere Positions

Telomeres

The ends of linear chromosomes are called **telomeres**. At the DNA level, these regions are distinguished by the presence of distinct nucleotide sequences repeated 50 to several hundred times. The repeated unit is usually 6–8 base pairs long and guanine-rich. Many vertebrates (including humans and mice) have the same repeat: 5'-TTAGGG-3'. Telomeres are composed of both single- and double-stranded DNA. Single-stranded DNA is found at the very end of the chromosome and is about 300 base pairs in length. It loops around to form a knot, held together by many telomere-associated proteins. This stabilizes the end of the chromosome; specialized telomere cap proteins distinguish telomeres from double-stranded breaks, and this prevents activation of repair pathways.

Telomeres function to prevent chromosome deterioration and also prevent fusion with neighboring chromosomes. They function as disposable buffers, blocking the ends of chromosomes. Since most prokaryotes have circular genomes, their DNA does not contain telomeres.

7.3 CHARACTERISTICS OF RNA

RNA is chemically distinct from DNA in three important ways:

1) RNA is **single-stranded**, except in some viruses.
2) RNA contains **uracil** instead of thymine.
3) The pentose ring in RNA is **ribose** rather than 2' deoxyribose.

As a result of this last difference, the RNA polymer is less stable, because the 2' hydroxyl can nucleophilically attack the backbone phosphate group of an RNA chain, causing hydrolysis when the remainder of the chain acts as leaving group. This cannot occur in DNA because there is no 2' hydroxyl. [Why is the stability of RNA relatively unimportant?[18] Anticancer drugs often seek to block growth of rapidly dividing cells by inhibiting production of thymine. Why is this an attractive target for cancer therapy?[19]] This chemical property has a big impact in molecular biology labs, where DNA samples are stable at a range of temperatures for a relatively long period of time, but high quality RNA is difficult to extract and is only stable for a short time.

There are several different types of RNA, each with a unique role.

Coding RNA

You are already familiar with **messenger RNA** (mRNA), the only type of coding RNA. This molecule carries genetic information to the ribosome, where it can be translated into protein (more information about translation can be found in *MCAT Biology Review*).

---

[18] Because a cell's DNA is necessary for the cell's entire life. RNA is a transient molecule that is transcribed, translated, and destroyed. As a matter of fact, the reason RNA contains uracil also has to do with the reduced need for fidelity in transcription as compared to replication. Without getting into the details, thymine is easier for DNA repair systems to work with, while uracil is much less energy-costly to make. So RNA has uracil, DNA has thymine.

[19] All cells require RNA production, even if they are not growing, in order to continually replenish degraded RNA. RNA contains the bases cytosine, guanine, uracil, and adenine, but only DNA contains thymine. Thus, if thymine production is blocked, only DNA *replication* will be inhibited and only rapidly dividing cells such as cancer cells will be affected. Unfortunately, some normal cells in the body normally divide a lot (such as lining cells of the gut and hair follicles), explaining the side effects of chemotherapy.

Messenger RNA is constantly produced and degraded, according to the cell's need for the protein encoded by each piece of mRNA. In fact, this is the principal means by which cells regulate the amount of each particular protein they synthesize. Note that in eukaryotes, the first RNA transcribed from DNA is an immature or precursor to mRNA called **heterogeneous nuclear RNA** (hnRNA). Processing events (such as addition of a cap and tail and splicing) are required for hnRNA to become mature mRNA. Since prokaryotes do not process their primary transcripts, hnRNA is found only in eukaryotes.

Non-Coding RNA

Non-coding RNA (ncRNA) is a functional RNA that is not translated into a protein. The human genome codes for thousands of ncRNAs, and there are several types. The two major types to know for the MCAT are transfer RNA (tRNA) and ribosomal RNA (rRNA).

Transfer RNA (tRNA) is responsible for translating the genetic code. Transfer RNA carries amino acids from the cytoplasm to the ribosome to be added to a growing protein. The structure of tRNA and how it does its job is discussed in *MCAT Biology Review*. [Estimate how many different tRNAs there are.[20]]

Ribosomal RNA (rRNA) is the major component of the ribosome. Humans have only four different types of rRNA molecules (18S, 5.8S, 28S, and 5S), though almost all of the RNA made in a given cell is rRNA. All rRNAs serve as components of the ribosome, along with many polypeptide chains. One rRNA provides the catalytic function of the ribosome, which is a little odd. In most other cases, enzymes are made from polypeptides. Catalytic RNAs are also called **ribozymes** (or ribonucleic acid enzymes), since they are capable of performing specific biochemical reactions, similar to protein enzymes.

Some other interesting non-coding RNAs include the following:

- **Small nuclear RNA** (snRNA) molecules (150 nucleotides) associate with proteins to form snRNP (small nuclear ribonucleic particles) complexes in the spliceosome.
- **MicroRNA** (miRNA) and **small interfering RNA** (siRNA) function in RNA interference (RNAi), a form of post-transcriptional regulation of gene expression. Both can bind specific mRNA molecules to either increase or decrease translation.
- **Long ncRNAs** are longer than 200 nucleotides. They help control the basal transcription level in a cell by regulating initiation complex assembly on promoters. They also contribute to many types of post-transcriptional regulation, by controlling splicing and translation, and they function in imprinting and X-chromosome inactivation.

---

[20] Each tRNA must recognize a codon on mRNA and respond by delivering the appropriate amino acid to the ribosome. There are 20 different amino acids, so there at least 20 different tRNAs. However, there are 61 possible codons, so there could be as many as 61 different tRNAs. The actual number is between 20 and 61, because the third nucleotide of the codon is often not needed for specificity of the amino acid.

Chapter 7 Summary

- DNA is the fundamental unit of inheritance in cells.

- DNA and RNA are polymers, made of nucleotide monomers. A nucleotide contains phosphate group(s), a sugar (either deoxyribose for DNA or ribose for RNA), and a nitrogenous base, either a purine (adenine or guanine) or a pyrimidine (thymine, cytosine, or uracil).

- In DNA, adenine always pairs with thymine via two hydrogen bonds, and cytosine always pairs with guanine via three hydrogen bonds.

- Uracil replaces thymine in RNA, and the ribose in RNA has an OH group on carbon 2.

- DNA is supercoiled in prokaryotes and packaged around histone proteins in eukaryotes.

- Eukaryotic DNA is divided into several linear chromosomes which have unique structures including the long (q) and short (p) arms, centromere and telomeres on the ends.

- There are several types of RNA that do not encode proteins. Some are directly involved in translation (rRNA and tRNA), while others play a role in gene expression (snRNA, miRNA, siRNA).

CHAPTER 7 FREESTANDING PRACTICE QUESTIONS

1. A chromosome in metaphase is stained to look for patterns in gene expression. Both light and dark regions on the chromosome appear. All of the following are true of the lightly stained region EXCEPT that:

A) it is likely to contain genes that are being actively transcribed.
B) it is called euchromatin, and is densely wrapped around histone proteins.
C) it contains an octamer of histones, composed of 2 units each of H2A, H2B, H3 and H4.
D) it consists of double-helical DNA bound by a single histone between nucleosomes.

2. Why is the 2′ OH group removed from ribose in order to form the monosaccharide component of DNA?

A) It ensures proper purine-purine pairing.
B) It converts a nucleoside into a nucleotide.
C) It sets up a phosphodiester bond.
D) It creates greater stability in the molecule.

3. High temperatures and some chemicals can separate (denature) two strands of antiparallel, complementary DNA. Which of the following accounts for the separation of double-stranded DNA after applying heat?

A) Disruption of the hydrogen bonds between pyrimidines and purines
B) Breakage of the phosphodiester bond between pyrimidines and purines
C) Disruption of the antiparallel nature of DNA strands
D) Disturbance in the hydrophobic forces between bases

4. Which of the following accurately describes the function of the centromere?

A) It is an attachment point for the synaptonemal complex during mitosis.
B) It is a cytoplasmic organelle that serves as an organizing center for microtubules.
C) It directly binds homologous chromosomes during meiosis.
D) It is an attachment point for spindle fibers via kinetochores.

5. DNA helicase is an enzyme that uses ATP to separate two complementary DNA strands during the replication process. Which of the following strands of DNA would require the most energy to separate from its complementary strand?

A) ATATATATAT
B) CCCGTAAAAT
C) CCGGCGTATA
D) ATCGATCGAT

6. What is a defining characteristic of heterogeneous nuclear RNA (hnRNA)?

A) It has a methylated guanine cap on the 5′ end.
B) It has a sequence containing introns and exons.
C) It contains uracil.
D) It has a poly A sequence on the 3′ end.

7. Shelterin is a protein complex involved in stabilizing the loop formed by the last approximately 300 bp of DNA at the end of eukaryotic chromosomes. A cell is found with mutations in the genes that code for shelterin. The most likely direct effect(s) of these mutations would be:

   I. activation of DNA repair pathways due to exposure of single-stranded DNA.
   II. an increase in double-stranded TTAGGG repeats.
   III. deletion of genes in the telomere regions.

A) I only
B) II and III only
C) I and III only
D) I, II and III

CHAPTER 7 PRACTICE PASSAGE

Antibiotic resistance presents an increasingly concerning problem for infectious disease management around the world. Perhaps one of the more disappointing recent trends is an increase in resistance to fluoroquinolone antibiotics. Well-tolerated with a minimal side effect profile, drugs from this class have been widely-prescribed for numerous infections, ranging from pneumonias to urinary tract infections. The main action of this class drug focuses on inhibiting DNA gyrase, an enzyme found in bacteria, but not humans. More specifically, the mechanism of action focuses on disruption of DNA replication by inhibiting the DNA topoisomerase II gyrase and ligase domains, while leaving nuclease activity intact. Acquisition of resistance to fluoroquinolones is typically associated with mutations, leading to structural changes in these proteins, increased expression of porins associated with decreased drug accumulation, as well as genes encoding peptides that directly block fluoroquinolone action.

In bacteria, gyrase utilizes the energy from ATP hydrolysis to relieve strain on the DNA double helix, while helicase unwinds it. The enzyme accomplishes this goal by generating double-stranded breaks with subsequent chiral wrapping of the strands to form a negative supercoil. Gyrase also relaxes any positive supercoils, allowing for unidirectional coiling across the whole DNA strand. Positive supercoiling is characterized by additional twisting and coiling in the same direction as the helix, whereas negative supercoiling are twists in the opposite direction. When able to bind to DNA topoisomerase II, fluoroquinolones disrupt these functions, resulting in the accumulation of positive supercoiling and increased strain on the DNA strand. Similarly, additional inhibition of the ligase domain by fluoroquinolones prevents DNA topoisomerase from repairing any breaks, further compromising the structure of the double-stranded molecule.

The structure of DNA gyrase consists of an A_2B_2 tetramer whose A and B subunits are encoded by the *gyrA* and *gyrB* genes. Generally speaking, the A subunit is responsible for inducing double-stranded breaks, while the B subunit facilitates the ATPase activity. Shown in Figure 1, the general mechanism of action by which supercoiling is induced involves creating a break in the first DNA strand (G) by forming a transient "gate" through which the second (T) strand can be "transported." It is generally accepted that fluoroquinolones inhibit DNA gyrase activity directly by forming a ternary complex with the enzyme that stabilizes it and prevents it from religating the broken DNA strands. The resulting fragmentation of chromosomal DNA ultimately leads to cell death.

Figure 1 Schematic of DNA gyrase structure and function

Microbiologists examining the genetic origins of fluoroquinolone resistance in *Mycobacterium tuberculosis* looked at the relative effect of multiple different mutations in the *gyrA* and *gyrB* genes on (1) the minimum inhibitory concentration (MIC) and (2) the resistance to ofloxacin, a second generation fluoroquinolone. The data pertaining to one potentially important instance are shown in Table 1.

gyrA mutation	*gyrB* mutation	MIC (mg/L)	Susceptibility
D89N	None	5	Resistant
None	N533T	1	Susceptible
None	None	4	Resistant

Table 1 Select MIC and susceptibility data for mutant and wild-type *Mycobacterium tuberculosis*

The MIC is characterized as the lowest concentration of antibiotic that will inhibit measurable bacterial growth after incubation.

Adapted from: Fabrega, A., et al. *Mechanism of action of and resistance to quinolones* and van Groll, A., et al. *Fluoroquinolone resistance in Mycobacterium tuberculosis and mutations in gyrA and gyrB.*

1. Which of the following bonds in DNA is the most likely target of DNA gyrase?

A) Hydrogen bond between aromatic bases
B) 5′–3′ phosphodiester bond between nucleotides
C) 4′ C–O covalent bond in deoxyribose
D) 1′ C–N covalent bond between deoxyribose and base

2. Based on information presented in the passage, which of the following statements is most likely to be true?

A) The hydrolysis of ATP is required to cut and religate the DNA double helix.
B) The toxicity of fluoroquinolones in humans is likely to be high due to an increased number of double-stranded breaks resulting from inhibition of DNA gyrase activity.
C) The formation of chromatin in bacteria is likely to be inhibited by fluoroquinolones due to characteristic disruption of orderly supercoiling.
D) The overall efficiency with which DNA is stored in the bacterial genome is disrupted by the action of fluoroquinolone antibiotics.

3. Which of the following is LEAST likely to be a driver of fluoroquinolone resistance in bacteria?

A) Adaptation characterized by increased expression of cell membrane efflux pumps
B) Mutations that lead to downregulation of the nuclease activity of topoisomerase
C) Mutations inducing structural changes in DNA gyrase
D) Transmission of code for direct fluoroquinolone inhibitor protein by plasmid

4. Which of the following conclusions is NOT supported by the data shown in Table 1?

A) Structural changes in any of the *gyr* genes result in increased fluoroquinolone resistance.
B) D89N mutation in the *gyrA* gene may result in a structural change that prevents fluoroquinolone binding.
C) N533T mutation in the *gyrB* gene may result in a structural change that further stabilizes the gyrase-DNA complex.
D) Not all mutations in the *gyr* genes result in increased fluoroquinolone resistance.

5. Which of the following graphs most accurately represents the effects of fluoroquinolones with increasing drug concentration?

A)

B)

C)

D)

SOLUTIONS TO CHAPTER 7 FREESTANDING PRACTICE QUESTIONS

1. **B** Make sure to highlight the word "EXCEPT" and write "A B C D" on your noteboard. Then evaluate each answer choice, writing "T" if it is true or "F" if it is false. The lightly stained regions of the chromosome are called euchromatin, which is thought to contain genes that are being actively transcribed into RNA (write "T" next to "A" on the noteboard). This is because the DNA is loosely wrapped around histone proteins, making it more accessible for transcription machinery (write "F" next to "B" on the noteboard). Chromatin is wrapped around eight histone proteins (write "T" next to "C" on the noteboard), called a nucleosome, and is punctuated by regions of ds-DNA between each nucleosome (write "T" next to "D" on the noteboard). Since choice B stands out with an "F" instead of a "T", it is the correct answer choice.

2. **D** Using deoxyribose (a ribose with the 2′ OH removed) generates greater stability in DNA, which is important because DNA, rather than RNA, is the primary form of long-term storage for genomes; certain viruses are a notable exception (choice D is correct). The OH group is not involved in base pairing, and, in any case, purines are meant to pair with pyrimidines (choice A is wrong). A nucleoside becomes a nucleotide when the phosphate is attached (choice B is wrong). The phosphodiester bond is formed between nucleotides using the phosphate backbone, not the 2′ OH group (choice C is wrong).

3. **A** Two strands of antiparallel and complementary DNA are held together in a helix by hydrogen bonding between pyrimidines and purines. As per the question stem, high temperatures can lead to the separation of strands, therefore the disruption of the hydrogen bonds. Phosphodiester bonds hold together the nucleotide backbone in a single strand of DNA, and are broken by nucleases rather than heat (choice B is wrong). Heat would not affect the propensity for a 5′-3′ DNA strands to bind with a complementary strand in 3′-5′ orientation (choice C is wrong). While heat does affect hydrophobic forces between bases, these forces serve to stabilize the DNA double helix, rather than directly bind the two strands together (choice D is wrong).

4. **D** The centromere is a region on the chromosome between sister chromatids. The synaptonemal complex is formed during meiosis, when there is pairing of homologous chromosomes, not mitosis (choice A is wrong). The cytoplasmic organelle that serves as an organizing center for microtubules is the centrosome, made up of two centrioles, not the centromere (choice B is false). Pairs of homologous chromosomes are held together by the synaptonemal complex proteins that anchor to the centromere, rather than the centromere binding the pairs directly (choice C is false). Centromeres serve as an attachment point for spindle fibers to mediate cell division (choice D is correct).

5. **C** There are three hydrogen bonds between cytosine (C) and guanine (G) base pairs, and only two hydrogen bonds between adenine (A) and thymine (T) pairs. Thus the strand with the most C:G base pairs will require the most energy to separate it from its complementary strand (choices A, B and D are incorrect; choice C is the answer).

6. **B** Heterogeneous nuclear RNA (hnRNA) is a precursor to mature RNA sequences that have had introns removed and exons spliced together; thus it can contain both types of sequence (choice B is correct). The presence of a methylated guanine cap indicates a fully modified transcript (choice A is wrong), as does the presence of poly-A tail (choice D is wrong). Uracil is a nucleotide used in all types of RNA and is not specific to hnRNA (choice C is wrong).

7. **A** Since this is a Roman numeral question, start by analyzing the Roman numeral item that appears in exactly two answer choices (in this case Item II); whether it is true or false you can eliminate half the answers. Item II is false: while telomere regions do contain TTAGGG repeats, active telomerase is responsible for adding these nucleotides. Not all cells express telomerase, and in any case this would not be affected by mutations shelterin (choices B and D can be eliminated). Since both remaining answer choices include Item I, it must be true and you can focus on Item III. Item III is false: there are no genes in the telomere regions, just many repeats of TTAGGG (choice C can be eliminated and choice A is correct). Note that Item I is in fact true: the very end segment of eukaryotic telomeres contains single-stranded DNA that forms a loop, which is stabilized by shelterin proteins, as per the question stem. If the shelterin complex is disrupted, it is likely that DNA repair pathways would be activated due to exposure of single-stranded DNA.

SOLUTIONS TO CHAPTER 7 PRACTICE PASSAGE

1. **B** The transient double-stranded breaks introduced by DNA gyrase involve the phosphodiester bonds that comprise the linkage between nucleotides. The breakage of none of the other bonds included in the answer choices would allow for one double helix to "pass through" another, as shown in Figure 1 (choice B is correct). Since the two strands of the double helix are not being separated, hydrogen bonds between bases will not be affected (choice A is wrong). Breakages of a single covalent bond within the deoxyribose ring or between deoxyribose and a base would not only be difficult and likely energetically unfavorable, it also wouldn't allow for the creation of the "gate" needed for DNA gyrase function (choices C and D are wrong).

2. **D** One major impact on the bacterial genome caused by the introduction of fluoroquinolones is the disruption of the uniform, orderly supercoiling process described in the passage; because this process is essential for efficient packaging and storage of bacterial DNA, its disruption would certainly reduce efficiency of storage of DNA in the bacterial genome (choice D is correct). As shown in Figure 1, hydrolysis of ATP comes after the helices have been cut and religated; the energy from ATP hydrolysis is most likely used to "reset" the enzyme to its original state after it has accomplished the cut/ligate action (choice A is wrong). Though there are some side effects in humans associated with fluoroquinolone administration, the main action of fluoroquinolone antibiotics focuses on disrupting the function of DNA gyrase, an enzyme not found in humans (choice B is wrong). Bacterial DNA is stored in the form of supercoiled circular DNA molecules, not the more complex chromatin-histone complexes found in eukaryotes (choice C is wrong).

3. **B** The increased expression of efflux pumps would likely reduce the intracellular concentration of an antibiotic, reducing its effect on gyrase activity and driving resistance (choice A is a driver of resistance and can be eliminated). The passage states that mutations in the code for DNA gyrase that result in structural alterations can lead to fluoroquinolone resistance (choice C is a driver in resistance and can be eliminated). Transmission of genetic code via plasmid is a commonly cited mechanism for transferring adaptive characteristics in bacteria (choice D is a driver of resistance and can be eliminated). However, simply downregulating the nuclease activity of DNA topoisomerase is unlikely to affect resistance. There is no reason to assume the drug can't bind just because the activity of the enzyme is slowed (choice B is least likely to drive resistance and is the correct answer).

4. **A** The data presented in Table 1 provides an important example that not all mutations in the *gyr* genes result in fluoroquinolone resistance; the *gyrB* mutation shown may actually increase susceptibility of the strain tested (choice A is not supported by the data and is the correct answer choice). While the increase in MIC for the D89N mutated strain is modest (5 mg/L) with respect to that for the non-mutated strain (4 mg/L), it is certainly possible that this mutation prevents fluoroquinolone binding. If the drug can't bind, the organism would be resistant (choice B is supported and can be eliminated). The passage states that fluoroquinolones stabilize the DNA-gyrase complex, and the table shows that the N533T mutation leads to a relative decrease in MIC, indicating increased susceptibility to the drug. Thus, it might be concluded that this mutation helps to stabilize the complex, thereby helping the action of the fluoroquinolones (choice C is supported and can be eliminated). This data does support the conclusion that not all mutations in *gyr* genes confer fluoroquinolone resistance; based on this data alone, it appears that some mutations may actually increase susceptibility (choice D is supported and can be eliminated).

5. **C** The passage states that fluoroquinolones disrupt the ability of DNA gyrase to introduce negative supercoils; therefore, the number of negative supercoils should decrease (choices B and D can be eliminated). This would lead to an accumulation of positive supercoils (choice A can be eliminated, and choice C is correct).

A HIGHLY DURABLE RNAi THERAPEUTIC INHIBITOR OF PCSK9

Kevin Fitzgerald, Ph.D., Suellen White, B.S.N., Anna Borodovsky, Ph.D., Brian R. Bettencourt, Ph.D., Andrew Strahs, Ph.D., Valerie Clausen, Ph.D., Peter Wijngaard, Ph.D., Jay D. Horton, M.D., Jorg Taubel, M.D., Ashley Brooks, M.B., Ch.B., Chamikara Fernando, M.B., B.S., Robert S. Kauffman, M.D., Ph.D., David Kallend, M.D., Akshay Vaishnaw, M.D., and Amy Simon, M.D.

This article was published on November 13, 2016, at NEJM.org.

N Engl J Med 2017;376:41-51. DOI: 10.1056/NEJMoa1609243 Copyright © 2016 Massachusetts Medical Society.

An elevated level of low-density lipoprotein (LDL) cholesterol is a major risk factor for cardiovascular disease. Despite the use of statin therapy, alone or in combination with other lipid-lowering medications, many at-risk patients continue to have elevated levels of LDL cholesterol. Hence, there is a need for additional treatment options for lowering of the LDL cholesterol level to reduce cardiovascular risk.

Proprotein convertase subtilisin–kexin type 9 (PCSK9) is a recently identified but well-validated target for LDL cholesterol–lowering therapy. This serine protease, which is expressed and secreted into the bloodstream predominantly by the liver, binds LDL receptors both intracellularly and extracellularly and promotes the lysosomal degradation of these receptors in hepatocytes, thereby increasing the circulating LDL cholesterol levels. PCSK9 loss-of-function mutations are associated with low circulating LDL cholesterol levels and diminished cardiovascular risk with no apparent negative health consequences.

PCSK9-blocking antibodies, administered once or twice monthly, reduce circulating PCSK9 levels and lower LDL cholesterol levels. Preliminary data suggest that long-term treatment with such antibodies is associated with a lower incidence of cardiovascular events than placebo. However, PCSK9 antibodies have a short duration of effect, necessitating frequent subcutaneous injections.

A recently discovered means of decreasing PCSK9 levels is the administration of small interfering RNA (siRNA) molecules. The siRNA molecules engage the natural pathway of RNA interference (RNAi) by binding intracellularly to the RNA-induced silencing complex (RISC), enabling it to cleave messenger RNA (mRNA) molecules encoding PCSK9 specifically. The cleaved mRNA is degraded and thus unavailable for protein translation, which results in decreased levels of the PCSK9 protein. A single siRNA-bound RISC is catalytic and cleaves many transcripts. This characteristic may be important during use of statins, which are known to up-regulate the production of PCSK9, potentially limiting the effectiveness of the drugs. The lipid nanoparticle ALN-PCS, an intravenous formulation of siRNA that inhibits PCSK9 synthesis, has been shown in a small phase 1 study to reduce the levels of both PCSK9 and LDL cholesterol in adult volunteers.

Inclisiran (ALN-PCSsc) is a long-acting, subcutaneously delivered, synthetic siRNA directed against PCSK9 that is conjugated to triantennary N-acetylgalactosamine carbohydrates. These carbohydrates bind to abundant liver-expressed asialoglycoprotein receptors, leading to inclisiran uptake specifically into hepatocytes. The siRNA was modified with a combination of phosphorothioate, 2'-O-methyl nucleotide, and 2'-fluoronucleotide modifications to improve molecular stability. In preclinical studies involving nonhuman primates, doses of more than 3 mg per kilogram of body weight resulted in reductions of more than 80% in plasma PCSK9 levels and approximately 60% lowering of the serum LDL cholesterol level, with peak effects lasting more than 30 days, with a very slow return to baseline levels over a period of 90 to 120 days after administration (unpublished data). This phase 1 study assessed the safety, side-effect profile, and pharmacodynamic effects of inclisiran when it was administered subcutaneously in single or multiple doses in healthy volunteers who had an LDL cholesterol level of at least 100 mg per deciliter (2.60 mmol per liter) and in a small number of participants taking a stable dose of statin cotherapy.

METHODS

Study Design and Oversight

We conducted this randomized, single-blind, placebo-controlled study in two stages — a single-dose phase (with ascending doses for sequential cohorts of patients), followed by a multiple-dose phase.

The study was performed at two contract research sites in the United Kingdom (Richmond Pharmacology and Covance). Data were collected by the investigators and analyzed by Covance and Alnylam Pharmaceuticals.

Participants

Men and women (18 to 60 years of age in the single-dose phase and 18 to 75 years of age in the multiple-dose phase) who had a serum LDL cholesterol level of at least 100 mg per deciliter and a fasting triglyceride level of less than 400 mg per deciliter (4.5 mmol per liter) were eligible. Participants taking statin therapy had to have been receiving a stable statin dose and regimen for at least 30 days before screening and had to have no planned changes during the study. Participants were not specifically instructed to maintain a stable dietary pattern. Participants with a history of cardiovascular disease, cerebrovascular disease, or diabetes mellitus were excluded except for those who were taking statins; such patients could be enrolled if they had noninsulindependent diabetes mellitus or controlled hypertension.

Randomization and Study Treatment

In the single-dose phase, six cohorts (with four participants each) were included. Participants in each cohort were randomly assigned in a 3:1 ratio to receive a subcutaneous injection of either inclisiran at a dose of 25, 100, 300, 500, or 800 mg (two cohorts for the 800-mg dose) or placebo.

In the multiple-dose phase, the participants in six cohorts (with four to eight participants each) were randomly assigned in a 3:1 ratio with the use of block sizes of four to receive inclisiran or placebo. One cohort received a dose of 125 mg once per week for 4 weeks, one cohort received a dose of 250 mg once every 2 weeks for 4 weeks, two cohorts (one of which was receiving statin therapy) received a dose of 300 mg once per month for 2 months, and two cohorts (one of which was receiving statin therapy) received a dose of 500 mg once per month for 2 months.

In the two phases, the first dose was administered on the day of randomization (day 0). Inclisiran or placebo (administered in sterile 0.9% normal saline) was injected subcutaneously into one or more sites of the abdomen; dose volumes of more than 1.5 ml were administered in two to three injections of equal volume. Inclisiran was supplied at a dose of 200 mg per milliliter of sterile solution. Participants were unaware of the assigned treatment because of syringe masking. No participant was included in more than one cohort.

Evaluations

Participants were monitored as inpatients for 3 days, with day −1 considered to be the day before initial administration. Participants underwent randomization and treatment commenced on day 0. Participants were evaluated as outpatients for safety, side-effect profile, and pharmacodynamic end points at specified times throughout the study period (56 days for the single-dose phase, and ≤84 days for the multiple-dose phase). Pharmacodynamic end points were evaluated for an additional month after the completion of the safety and side-effect profile assessments.

Participants were considered to have completed the trial according to the protocol after their final planned safety and pharmacodynamic follow-up visit. If at that visit the most recent three LDL cholesterol levels averaged less than 80% of the baseline value, pharmacodynamic monitoring continued every 2 weeks for 1 month, and then every 4 weeks, until the more recent three LDL cholesterol measurements averaged 80% or more of the baseline value or until 180 days after the last dose of inclisiran or placebo, whichever came sooner.

The safety evaluation included clinical laboratory tests (hematologic, biochemical, coagulation, and urinalysis tests), vital signs (oral body temperature, blood pressure, heart rate, and respiration rate), physical examination, 12-lead electrocardiography (ECG), and adverse-event monitoring.

Pharmacodynamic monitoring included plasma PCSK9 and serum LDL cholesterol measurements. The exploratory biomarkers that were evaluated included levels of total cholesterol, high-density lipoprotein (HDL) cholesterol, non-HDL cholesterol (total cholesterol level minus the HDL cholesterol level), apolipoprotein B, lipoprotein(a), and triglycerides.

Statistical Analysis

In each study phase, data from the participants in the placebo group were combined across cohorts for analysis. The mean percent reductions in the plasma PCSK9 level, as compared with baseline, at day 84 after the first dose of the study regimen were compared with those in the placebo group by means of a repeated-measures analysis of covariance (ANCOVA), including the baseline PCSK9 level as a covariate, and treatment-by-time interaction. The model used an autoregressive first-order covariance structure. This method was also used for the lipid data. A nominal P value of less than 0.05 was considered to indicate statistical significance.

RESULTS

Participants

The characteristics of the participants at baseline, according to study phase and assigned group, in the safety population are shown in Table 1.

Safety and Side-Effect Profile

All the adverse events were mild or moderate (grade 1 or 2) in severity. There were no treatment discontinuations that were due to adverse events, and no serious adverse events were reported.

PCSK9 Levels

In the single-dose phase, inclisiran at a dose of 300 mg or more was associated with reductions from baseline in the PCSK9 level that were significant, as compared with placebo, at day 84 (Table 2 and Fig. 1A). The magnitudes of the reduction in the PCSK9 level were similar across the dose range of 300 to 800 mg (least-squares mean change, 69.9 to 74.5%); the largest reduction, 74.5%, occurred in the group that was treated with 300 mg of inclisiran. PCSK9 levels had returned to baseline values by day 180 after the receipt of the dose in the 25-mg and 100-mg cohorts. For inclisiran doses of 300 mg or more, the PCSK9 levels remained reduced, as compared with baseline, at day 180 after receipt of the dose (Fig. 1A).

In the multiple-dose phase, all the inclisiran regimens were associated with reductions from baseline in the PCSK9 level that were significant, as compared with placebo, at day 84 after receipt of the first dose (Table 3 and Fig. 1B). The magnitude of the reductions in the PCSK9 level were similar across all the inclisiran cohorts, with the least-squares mean change from baseline ranging from 71.8 to 83.8% at day 84 after receipt of the first dose; the largest reduction, 83.8%, was observed in the group that received 500 mg of inclisiran once per month for 2 months as well as statin cotherapy. Levels of PCSK9 remained reduced, as compared with baseline, in all the inclisiran cohorts at day 196 after receipt of the first dose (Fig. 1B).

LDL Cholesterol Levels

In the single-dose phase, reductions from baseline in the LDL cholesterol level that were significant, as compared with placebo, were observed at day 84 after receipt of inclisiran doses of 100 mg or more (Table 2 and Fig. 2A). At these doses, the least-squares mean reductions in the LDL cholesterol level ranged from 36.7 to 50.6%; the largest reduction, 50.6%, was observed in the group that received 500 mg of inclisiran. The LDL cholesterol levels returned toward baseline values at 180 days after receipt of the dose in the 25-mg and 100-mg cohorts, whereas the levels remained reduced, as compared with baseline, until at least 180 days after receipt of inclisiran doses of 300 mg or more (Fig. 2A).

In the multiple-dose phase, reductions in the LDL cholesterol level that were significant, as compared with placebo, were observed at day 84 after receipt of the first dose for all inclisiran regimens except for the cohort that received 125 mg weekly for 4 weeks. Reductions ranged from a least-squares mean change of 45.1 to 59.7%, with the largest reduction, 59.7%, occurring in the group that received 300 mg of inclisiran monthly for 2 months (Table 3 and Fig. 2B). The LDL cholesterol levels remained reduced, as compared with baseline, in all the inclisiran cohorts at day 196 after receipt of the first dose (Fig. 2B).

Exploratory Analyses

In both the single-dose and multiple-dose phases, decreases in the levels of total cholesterol, non-HDL cholesterol, and apolipoprotein B were noted in participants treated with inclisiran (Tables 2 and 3). The reductions in these variables from baseline to day 84 after receipt of the first dose were significant, as compared with placebo, for single or multiple doses of 250 mg or more.

Table 1   Demographic and Clinical Characteristics of the Participants at Baseline (Safety Population)*

| Characteristic | Single-Dose Phase | | Multiple-Dose Phase | | | |
| | | | Placebo | | Inclisiran | |
	Placebo (N = 6)	Inclisiran (N = 18)	with statin (N = 4)†	without statin (N = 8)	with statin (N = 9)‡	without statin (N = 24)
Age — yr	48 ± 14	46 ± 10	58 ± 3	51 ± 14	54 ± 16	51 ± 12
Male sex —no. (%)	2 (33)	17 (94)	2 (50)	6 (75)	4 (44)	17 (71)
Race —no. (%)						
White	4 (67)	12 (67)	4 (100)	7 (88)	6 (67)	19 (79)
Other	2 (33)	6 (33)	0	1 (12)	3 (33)	5 (21)
Weight —kg	70.6 ± 12.0	77.1 ± 7.7	74.3 ± 5.1	77.6 ± 10.3	77.7 ± 17.0	74.7 ± 11.7
Height —cm	168 ± 11	173 ± 6	168 ± 10	171 ± 9	171 ± 12	171 ± 8
LDL cholesterol —mg/dl	131.5 ± 19.3	163.0 ± 32.9	143.1 ± 89.7	131.5 ± 20.9	143.4 ± 29.8	139.3 ± 32.3
Triglycerides —mg/dl	70.9 ± 12.4	135.5 ± 55.7	150.6 ± 46.9	124.0 ± 38.1	116.3 ± 64.3	123.4 ± 82.9
PCSK9 —μg/liter	279.0 ± 99.5	275.4 ± 58.2	460.7 ± 56.3	276.2 ± 58.7	451.8 ± 132.2	317.1 ± 66.8

* Plus–minus values are means ±SD.

† Three participants were taking simvastatin at a dose of 40 mg per day, and one was taking pravastatin at a dose of 20 mg per day.

‡ Four participants were taking atorvastatin at a dose of 40 mg per day, two at a dose of 20 mg per day, and one at a dose of 10 mg per day; one participant was taking simvastatin at a dose of 40 mg per day and one at a dose of 20 mg per day.

Table 2   Least-Squares Mean Percent Change from Baseline in Pharmacodynamic Variables at Day 84 in the Single-Dose Phase (Pharmacodynamic Population)*

| Variable | Placebo (N = 6) | Inclisiran | | | | |
		25 mg (N = 3)	100 mg (N = 3)	300 mg (N = 3)	500 mg (N = 3)	800 mg (N = 6)
PCSK9						
Percent change (95% CI)	0.6 (−24.2 to 30.4)	46.6 (−65.4 to −17.8)†	32.0 (−52.5 to −2.7)	74.5 (−82.1 to −63.6)‡	69.9 (−78.9 to −57.0)‡	73.1 (−79.1 to −65.4)‡
LDL cholesterol						
Percent change (95% CI)	10.9 (−26.0 to 7.1)	21.5 (−41.3 to 5.0)	36.7 (−50.2 to −19.4)†	50.0 (−60.7 to −36.3)‡	50.6 (−61.3 to −36.9)‡	43.4 (−52.5 to −32.4)‡
Total cholesterol						
Percent change (95% CI)	4.4 (−15.9 to 8.7)	12.0 (−30.1 to 10.8)	17.7 (−30.0 to −3.4)	30.9 (−41.2 to −18.9)¶	27.1 (−38.2 to −14.0)†	29.1 (−36.8 to −20.6)¶
HDL cholesterol						
Percent change (95% CI)	13.6 (−9.2 to 42.1)	7.3 (−22.0 to 47.7)	17.9 (−9.2 to 53.1)	36.8 (2.9 to 82.0)	7.4 (−17.4 to 39.8)	0.1 (−16.8 to 20.5)
Non-HDL cholesterol						
Percent change (95% CI)	11.7 (−23.7 to 2.3)	19.8 (−36.1 to 0.6)	28.4 (−40.8 to −13.5)	48.9 (−57.8 to −38.2)‡	36.3 (−47.4 to −22.9)¶	37.0 (−44.9 to −28.0)¶
Apolipoprotein B						
Percent change (95% CI)	15.3 (−31.4 to 4.6)	11.3 (−36.8 to 24.5)	26.5 (−43.3 to −4.7)	47.1 (−59.0 to −31.9)¶	39.9 (−53.9 to −21.7)†	37.5 (−47.7 to −25.2)†
Lipoprotein (a)						
Percent change (95% CI)	3.6 (−28.6 to 50.2)	14.0 (−55.1 to 64.6)	20.8 (−51.0 to 28.0)	44.5 (−65.7 to −10.4)†	35.5 (−60.1 to 4.3)	21.3 (−45.0 to 12.6)

Differences shown in the inclisiran groups are with the placebo group. CI denotes confidence interval, and HDL high-density lipoprotein.

† P<0.05 for the pairwise comparison with placebo.

‡ P<0.001 for the pairwise comparison with placebo.

§ The group nadir was defined as the largest mean percent reduction from the baseline value during the study.

¶ P < 0.01 for the pairwise comparison with placebo.

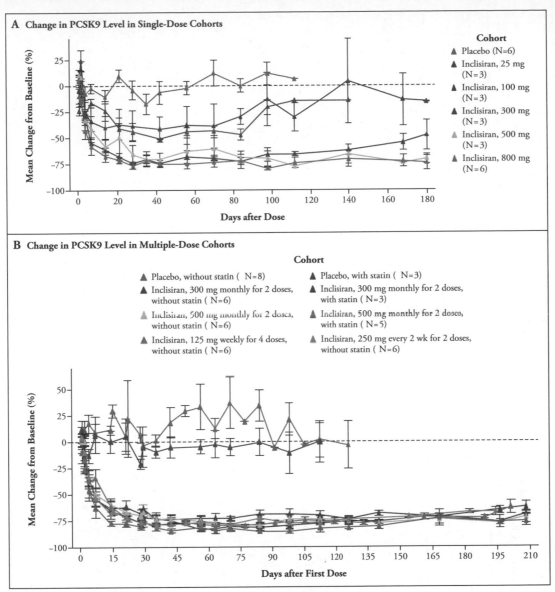

Figure 1. Change in Plasma Levels of Proprotein Convertase Subtilisin–Kexin Type 9 (PCSK9), According to Study Group and Dose Cohort. Shown are the effects (mean percentage changes from baseline) of single or multiple doses of inclisiran or placebo on plasma levels of PCSK9 over time. Baseline values were the average of all the study measurements obtained before the first dose.

Table 3 Least-Squares Mean Percent Change from Baseline in Pharmacodynamic Variables at Day 84 after the First Dose in the Multiple-Dose Phase (Pharmacodynamic Population)*

Variable	Placebo (N = 11)	Inclisiran					
		300 mg with Statin (N = 3)	300 mg without Statin (N = 6)	500 mg with Statin (N = 5)	500 mg without Statin (N = 6)	125 mg without Statin (N = 6)	250 mg without Statin (N = 6)
PCSK9							
Percent change (95% CI)	16.9 (−2.4 to 40.0)	−79.9 (−85.4 to −72.5)†	−71.8 (−77.4 to −64.8)†	−83.8 (−87.3 to −79.3)†	−81.5 (−85.2 to −76.9)†	−77.4 (−81.9 to −71.8)†	−75.7 (−80.5 to −69.6)†
LDL cholesterol							
Percent change (95% CI)	−14.2 (−30.2 to 5.5)	−45.1 (−61.6 to −21.4)‡	−59.7 (−68.7 to −48.1)†	−53.2 (−64.5 to −38.3)§	−51.7 (−62.5 to −37.8)§	−39.8 (−51.1 to −25.9)	−52.2 (−62.9 to −38.4)§
Total cholesterol							
Percent change (95% CI)	−7.6 (−15.5 to 1.0)	−24.9 (−35.8 to −12.0)‡	−40.4 (−46.7 to −33.4)†	−30.4 (−38.4 to −21.3)†	−27.0 (−34.7 to −18.3)§	−23.8 (−31.9 to −14.7)	−34.5 (−41.4 to −26.7)†
HDL cholesterol							
Percent change (95% CI)	0.6 (−6.0 to 7.6)	10.8 (−1.5 to 24.6)	11.7 (2.7 to 21.4)	5.3 (−3.9 to 15.3)	12.8 (3.8 to 22.6)‡	12.9 (3.8 to 22.7)	12.9 (−4.2 to 13.1)
Non-HDL cholesterol							
Percent change (95% CI)	−10.6 (−21.3 to 1.6)	−35.7 (−48.7 to −19.3)‡	−56.9 (−63.3 to −49.4)†	−46.2 (−54.9 to −35.8)†	−45.1 (−53.3 to −35.5)†	−36.9 (−46.3 to −25.9)	−45.3 (−53.4 to −35.8)†
Apolipoprotein B							
Percent change (95% CI)	−12.8 (−23.2 to −1.0)	−37.2 (−49.8 to −21.4)‡	−52.4 (−59.4 to −44.2)†	−41.8 (−51.1 to −30.7)†	−46.4 (−54.3 to −37.2)†	−33.3 (−43.1 to −21.8)	−46.5 (−54.3 to −37.3)†
Lipoprotein (a)							
Percent change (95% CI)	−6.0 (−26.7 to 20.4)	−30.7 (−54.3 to 5.1)	−19.2 (−40.0 to 8.8)	−42.7 (−59.7 to −18.4)‡	−27.4 (−45.8 to −2.7)	−22.7 (−28.4 to −16.5)‡	−28.1 (−46.4 to −3.4)

Differences shown in the inclisiran groups are with the placebo group.
† P<0.001 for the pairwise comparison with placebo.
‡ P<0.05 for the pairwise comparison with placebo.
§ P<0.01 for the pairwise comparison with placebo.

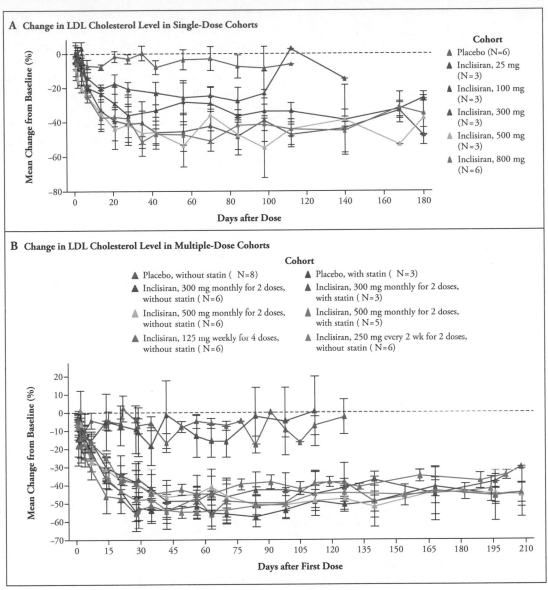

Figure 2. Effects on Serum Levels of Low-Density Lipoprotein (LDL) Cholesterol, According to Study Group and Dose Cohort. Shown are the effects (mean percentage changes from baseline) of inclisiran or placebo on the serum levels of LDL cholesterol over time. Baseline values were the average of all the study measurements taken before the first dose.

DISCUSSION

In this study, treatment with inclisiran, a subcutaneously administered RNAi therapeutic agent targeting PCSK9 to reduce LDL cholesterol levels, resulted in no treatment discontinuations due to adverse events and no serious adverse events at the doses we studied. All the adverse events were mild or moderate in severity.

Single doses of inclisiran of 300 mg or more and all the multiple-dose regimens that we studied were associated with reductions of circulating levels of both PCSK9 and LDL cholesterol at 84 days after receipt of the first dose. We observed reductions in the PCSK9 level of up to 83.8% and in the LDL cholesterol level of up to 59.7%. We also observed lowering of the serum LDL cholesterol level when inclisiran was administered to patients taking stable doses of statin therapy. These findings add to previous nonclinical and clinical evidence that supports the ability of RNAi therapeutic agents in general to inhibit the synthesis of liver-derived target proteins.

The results of this study also add to the clinical evidence from anti-PCSK9 antibody trials that supports PCSK9 as a therapeutic target for significant lowering of the LDL cholesterol level. The magnitude of the lowering of the LDL cholesterol level that we found with inclisiran was generally similar to that observed previously with anti-PCSK9 antibodies or intensive statin therapy. However, inclisiran differs mechanistically from anti-PCSK9 antibodies. Whereas anti-PCSK9 antibodies bind to extracellular PCSK9 (produced from any tissue) and prevent its interaction with the LDL receptor, inclisiran inhibits the synthesis of PCSK9 protein specifically in the liver.

The pharmacodynamic profile of inclisiran also differs substantially from that of the anti-PCSK9 antibodies that have been studied to date. The effect on the PCSK9 and LDL cholesterol levels persisted for at least 180 days after the initiation of treatment, with little variation over the 6-month period after the receipt of the first dose. Our data suggest that inclisiran has the potential to provide effective management of hypercholesterolemia with administration every 3 or 6 months, as compared with the recommended regimens of administration once or twice monthly for the currently approved antibodies.

The limitations of the study should be considered carefully. First, although the trial was randomized and placebo-controlled, it was a singleblind trial and included only a limited number of participants in order to obtain an initial assessment of safety and pharmacodynamics. Therefore, the results must be regarded as preliminary and be confirmed in larger clinical trials of longer duration. Second, the sample included mainly healthy participants with relatively normal lipid profiles, albeit with a baseline LDL cholesterol level of at least 100 mg per deciliter. A limited number of patients taking statins were enrolled, and the coadministration of nonstatin LDL cholesterol–lowering agents was not investigated. In addition, in the multiple-dose phase, subsequent doses of inclisiran were administered well within the period of maximal pharmacodynamic activity of the first dose. Also, the cumulative doses of the multiple-dose regimens (500 to 1000 mg) were similar to the most effective single doses studied (300 to 800 mg). This situation may explain the apparently moderate incremental effects of increasing doses on the levels of PCSK9 and LDL cholesterol.

In conclusion, in this small phase 1 study, single or multiple doses of inclisiran, an RNAi therapeutic agent targeting PCSK9, were administered over a 1-month period. No serious adverse events occurred, and consistent, sustained reductions in the circulating PCSK9 and LDL cholesterol levels were observed.

JOURNAL ARTICLE EXERCISE 3

The science sections on the MCAT include a significant number of passages with experiments. Questions for these passages often ask you to analyze data, read charts and graphs, and come to some reasonable conclusion based on the information they give you. If you don't know how to extract information efficiently and analyze data effectively, you will be at a distinct disadvantage.

There are three "Journal Article Exercises" in this book. In this final exercise, you'll read and extract information from the article and then complete an MCAT passage based on this article. After that, we'll show you the "correct" information to pull out and the answers to the passage.

As before, when analyzing an experiment, you should be able to:

- identify the control group(s).
- extract information from graphs and data tables.
- determine how the experimental group(s) change relative to the control.
- determine if the results are statistically significant.
- come to a reasonable conclusion about WHY the results were observed.
- consider potential weaknesses in the study.
- determine how to increase the power of the study.
- decide what the next most logical experiment or study should be.

And, as before, the goal of these exercises is NOT to learn content from the articles, just to get a little more comfortable reading and extracting information from them.

For the (abridged) article pages 211–218. summarize the purpose of the experiment and the methods in a few sentences. Remember the mnemonic: Oh ouR Car Won't Start (ORCWS).

- O = Organism and Organization
- R = Results
- C = Control and Comparison
- W = Weirdness
- S = Statistics

Try interpreting the data on your own before reading the results/discussion section. When you do read the discussion, consider:

- What are the conclusions of the study?
- How are the conclusions supported by the data?
- What potential weaknesses or flaws do you see in the experimental design? Are these addressed in the discussion section?
- How might this study be potentially biased?
- How might this study be improved?
- What would be the next most logical experiment?

Answer these questions for the article on pages 211–218.

1. **O = Organism and Organization:**
   - Is the research being conducted on humans or on animals or on bacteria in a petri dish, or something else?

     _____

     _____

   - What is being done to these organisms?

     _____

     _____

   - Are there any unique qualities to these organisms?

     _____

     _____

   - Are there multiple groups?

     _____

     _____

   - Is the study conducted over a long period of time with multiple data points, or is it a short-term study?

     _____

     _____

   - Does it have a large or small n?

     _____

     _____

2. **R = Results:**
   - Where and how are the results presented? Is it a graph? A data table? Figures and images?

     _____

     _____

   - What is/are the independent variable(s)?

     _____

     _____

   - What is/are the dependent variable(s)?

     _____

     _____

   - What are the results of the study?

     _____

     _____

- Do the results show correlation or cause and effect, or both? Describe.

  _____

  _____

3. **C = Control and Comparison:**
   - Is there a control group?

     _____

     _____

   - How does it differ from the experimental group? Is it given a placebo or nothing at all? Is it held under different conditions?

     _____

     _____

   - If there are multiple experimental groups, how do they differ from one another?

     _____

     _____

   - Is it a blinded study? If so, double-blind or single-blind?

     _____

     _____

4. **W = Weirdness:**
   - Does anything or do any of the results stand out as unexpected?

     _____

     _____

5. **S = Statistics:**
   - Was any sort of statistical analysis done?

     _____

     _____

   - How is it presented? Are there error bars on a graph? Standard errors around a mean? Are there p-values? Is there an asterisk indicating statistical significance?

     _____

     _____

   - Is there any data that is not statistically significant?

     _____

     _____

6. **Interpreting the data:**
   - What are the conclusions of the study?

     _____

     _____

- How are the conclusions supported by the data?

  _____

  _____

- What potential weaknesses or flaws do you see in the experimental design? Are these addressed in the discussion section?

  _____

  _____

- How might this study be potentially biased?

  _____

  _____

- How might this study be improved?

  _____

  _____

- What would be the next most logical experiment?

  _____

  _____

7. **Final Summary of Experiment and Results:**

  _____

  _____

  _____

  _____

  _____

  _____

JOURNAL ARTICLE EXERCISE 3 PASSAGE

Low density lipoproteins (LDLs) transport cholesterol made by the liver to cells that require it as source material for steroid hormones, a component of cell plasma membranes, or other similar functions. However, elevated LDL levels, typically characterized as above 100 mg/dL, present a clinical risk; at these higher levels, additional circulating cholesterol carried by LDLs may become attached to the walls of blood vessels, both forming plaques and contributing to arteries becoming hardened as part of coronary artery disease.

Hepatocytes and other body cells have receptors that can bind LDLs to limit their distribution in the body. Those receptors can be destroyed by serine proteases; one example is proprotein convertase subtilisin–kexin type 9 (PCSK9), which triggers lysosomal degradation of LDL receptors. Therapeutic approaches to dealing with high LDL levels have sought to target the lipoprotein itself as well as enzymes like PCSK9 to help manage the overall lipid profile in the body.

A new therapeutic, inclisiran, acts as a small interfering RNA (siRNA) and is thought to limit expression of PCSK9. Researchers aimed to determine if administration of inclisiran lowered circulating levels of LDL, in part by helping to maintain the receptors that can bind it. A limited clinical trial of the drug was launched in which subjects were either given a single dose of inclisiran (N = 3 for each dose level), or a placebo (N = 6), then tracked for six months, or given two doses per month (or a placebo) and tracked for seven months. All subjects were tracked for several months. Those in the multidose group were also divided such that some participants in both the treatment and placebo groups were also given a statin, a class of drugs that helps remove cholesterol from plaques attached to blood vessels (N < 8 for all multidose groups). Measures of PCSK9 and LDL were taken throughout the study and results are presented in Figures 1 and 2.

Figure 1 Change in plasma levels of PCSK9 as mean percentage changes from baseline. All cohorts compared to placebo. At day 84, single-dose cohorts, $p < 0.001$; multiple-dose cohorts without statin, $p < 0.01$; multiple-dose cohorts with statin, $p < 0.001$.

Figure 2 Changes in serum levels of LDL cholesterol as mean percentage changes from baseline. All cohorts compared to placebo. At day 84, single-dose cohorts, $p < 0.001$; multiple-dose cohorts without statin, $p < 0.01$; multiple-dose cohorts with statin, $p < 0.001$.

Adapted from Fitzgerald, K., White, S., Borodovsky, A. *et al.* A Highly Durable RNAi Therapeutic Inhibitor of PCSK9. *N Engl J Med* **376** (2017).

1. Based on the experimental data at approximately two months, which treatment might be interpreted as most effective?

A) Multiple doses of placebo paired with a statin
B) Single 100 mg dose of inclisiran
C) Multiple 500 mg doses of inclisiran not paired with a statin
D) Multiple 500 mg doses of inclisiran paired with a statin

2. It is most likely that inclisiran will have what effect on treated cells?

A) RNA polymerase will be prevented from binding promoter sequences for the targeted genes.
B) Transcripts for the targeted genes will be broken down before they are translated.
C) Post-transcriptional modification will be prevented as methylated guanine is blocked from binding the 5′ end of the transcript.
D) The sense strand of the DNA helix will be transcribed instead of the anti-sense strand.

3. According to the data in Figures 1 and 2, what conclusion about PCSK9 and LDL is best suppported?

A) Compared to placebo, multiple doses of inclisiran with statin have a statistically significant effect on the level of PCSK9, but not on the level of LDL.
B) Statically speaking, multiple doses of inclisiran given without additional statin have the same effect on the level of PCSK9 and the level of LDL.
C) The single dose protocol of inclisiran only shows a statistically significant effect when paired with statin treatment.
D) Compared to placebo, the single dose protocol of inclisiran has a statistically significant effect on the level of PCSK9 and LDL.

4. If LDL levels remain above 100 mg/dL for an extended period, the amount of oxygen supplied to the cardiac muscle will:

A) decrease due to increased stiffness in coronary blood vessels and decreased flow due to plaque blockage.
B) decrease due to hardening in the vessels involved in external respiration in the lungs
C) increase due to the stabilizing effect produced with hardening of blood vessels.
D) increase due to a higher respiratory rate resulting from the stress of coronary artery disease.

5. Based on the available experimental data, what limitation is evident in the design of the protocol?

A) The small number of different doses of inclisiran that were included in both
B) Statins were not tested on their own
C) Small sample size (N) restricts the power of the experiment
D) Statistical analysis requires calculation of both p values and standard deviation

SOLUTIONS TO JOURNAL ARTICLE EXERCISE 3

1. **O = Organism and Organization:**
    *   Is the research being conducted on humans or on animals or on bacteria in a petri dish, or something else? *Humans (21 women, 48 men)*
    *   What is being done to these organisms? *They are being treated with either inclisiran (a drug) or a placebo to see if the drug will lower the levels of low density lipoproteins (LDLs).*
    *   Are there any unique qualities to these organisms? *A requirement for the study was subjects having an LDL level of 100 or higher.*
    *   Are there multiple groups? *Yes, one group receives inclisiran in a single dose, and one group receives inclisiran as a multidose process. The multidose group was also split into those receiving a statin drug versus those not taking a statin.*
    *   Is the study conducted over a long period of time with multiple data points, or is it a short-term study? *Long-ish. The single-dose group was followed for approximately six months while the multidose group was followed for approximately seven months.*
    *   Does it have a large or small *n*? *The n for the study is relatively small, but it is still reasonable given the challenges in recruiting human subjects.*

2. **R = Results:**
    *   Where and how are the results presented? Is it a graph? A data table? Figures and images? *The results are presented in tables and graphs.*
    *   What is/are the independent variable(s)? *Time, inclisiran versus placebo, statin versus no statin*
    *   What is/are the dependent variable(s)? *Measurement of LDL levels and proprotein convertase subtilisin–kexin type 9 (PCSK9), a serine protease that can raise LDL levels by destroying its receptors.*
    *   What are the results of the study? *Single-dose treatment with inclisiran generated a statistically significant reduction in LDL and PCSK9 at doses of 300 mg or higher as did each level of the multidose treatment protocol.*
    *   Do the results show correlation or cause and effect, or both? Describe. *The results are causative; both the single-dose and multidose versions of the protocol used a placebo group and the effect seen in those receiving inclisiran was not seen in the placebo subjects.*

3. **C = Control and Comparison:**
    *   Is there a control group? *Yes*
    *   How does it differ from the experimental group? Is it given a placebo or nothing at all? Is it held under different conditions? *Yes, both the single-dose and multidose groups have subsets of subjects receiving a placebo instead of inclisiran.*
    *   If there are multiple experimental groups, how do they differ from one another? *The single-dose group had one dose administered, the dose ranging from 25 mg to 800 mg. The multidose group had a smaller number of dose sizes being tested, but also included an additional variant as to whether or not the subject received a statin drug along with the inclisiran.*
    *   Is it a blinded study? If so, double blind or single blind? *Yes, single-blinded*

4. **W = Weirdness:**
   - Does anything or do any of the results stand out as unexpected? *The effectiveness of the single-dose protocol was demonstrated starting at 300 mg and for the multidose protocol, all doses were found to be effective, but the lowest total dose in the multidose protocol was 250 mg, which was less than the effective amount in the single-dose protocol.*

5. **S = Statistics:**
   - Was any sort of statistical analysis done? *Yes*
   - How is it presented? Are there error bars on a graph? Standard errors around a mean? Are there p-values? Is there an asterisk indicating statistical significance? *P-values, standard errors reported on means, error bars on graphs*
   - Is there any data that is not statistically significant? *The placebo branches for both the single-dose and multidose versions of the protocol did not have a statistically significant effect.*

6. **Interpreting the data:**
   - What are the conclusions of the study? *Treatment with inclisiran could be effective at reducing LDL levels for those with LDL levels above 100 mg per deciliter, with or without the accompanying use of a statin.*
   - How are the conclusions supported by the data? *The conclusions are supported based on the statistically significant drop both in the measure of LDL in treated groups as well as the drops in PCSK9.*
   - What potential weaknesses or flaws do you see in the experimental design? Are these addressed in the discussion section? *The protocol worked to recruit across a range of ages, but the study population was mostly male and mostly white. The number of subjects would need to be larger and their selection would need to represent a broader range of demographics.*
   - How might this study be potentially biased? *This study may be biased based on the composition of its patient population.*
   - How might this study be improved? *A larger N with a broader range of demographics represented*
   - What would be the next most logical experiment? *An additional trial with a larger pool of subjects run at more than two centers*

7. **Final Summary of Experiment and Results:**
   - *In this journal article, the effect of inclisiran on both LDL levels and the levels of PCSK9 (an enzyme that can cause elevations in LDL) was evaluated in a population with elevated LDL. Subjects were given either a single dose of the drug or a placebo, across a range of doses; some subjects received multiple doses across a smaller range of doses. The multidose group was split into those receiving a statin drug or not. All subjects receiving at least 300 mg in the single-dose trial, and all subjects in the multidose trial (starting at two doses of 125 mg), showed a significant decrease in both LDL and PCSK9.*

SOLUTIONS TO JOURNAL ARTICLE EXERCISE 3 PASSAGE

1. **D** Two months is approximately 60 days so examine that time point on each of the graphs. The placebo in all cases is less effective than any other treatment (choice A can be eliminated). A single 100 mg dose triggered an approximate 30% decrease in both measures; however, other treatment protocols available in the answer choices did better (choice B can be eliminated). Multiple doses at 500 mg but lacking a statin reduced PCSK9 levels by about 75% and LDL levels by about 40%, while multiple doses at 500 mg with a statin similarly lowered PCSK9 levels but reduced LDL levels even further (almost 60%; choice C can be eliminated and choice D is correct).

2. **B** The passage states that inclisiran as an siRNA; these trigger post-transcriptional destruction of mRNA transcripts, preventing them from being translated and preventing expression of the associated proteins (choice B is correct). siRNAs do not interact with the RNA polymerases (choice A is wrong) nor do they prevent binding of the 5' methylated guanine cap necessary for a transcript to continue with translation in eukaryotic cells (choice C is wrong). This form of RNA acts post-transcriptionally and does not change which strand of the DNA helix is transcribed in the first place (choice D is wrong).

3. **D** Since the graph captions contain information on p values, this would be the best source to assess statistical significance. The multidose protocol that includes statin has $p < 0.001$ for both PCSK9 and LDL, indicating that both effects are statistically significant (choice A is eliminated). The multidose protocol that does not include statin has a p value less than 0.001 for PCSK9, but less than 0.01 for LDL; while both are significant, they are not necessarily the same as each other (choice B is eliminated). The single dose protocol is not run with statin treatment, so this experimental group cannot be evaluated (choice C is eliminated). However, the single dose protocol has a p value less than 0.001 for both PCSK9 and LDL, showing statistical significance for both (choice D is correct).

4. **A** The passage describes LDL levels above 100 mg/dL as a clinical concern due to the increased level of plaques found in blood vessels and their link to coronary artery disease. Blocking these vessels would physically limit oxygenated blood flow (choices C and D can be eliminated). The passage states that arteries (the vessels delivering oxygen to the heart) are hardened, not the capillary beds around the lungs where external respiration occurs (choice B can be eliminated and choice A is correct).

5. **C** The graphs report on the number of subjects in each treatment arm and these numbers are fairly small; this will limit the power of the study overall (choice C is correct). There is a range of doses represented and not enough information is present to evaluate whether this is sufficient or if there really should be more; without more support, this cannot be evaluated (choice A can be eliminated). The statins are tested on their own; the multidose cohorts include a group that was administered a placebo plus statin, effectively testing the statin on its own (choice B can be eliminated). Standard deviation analysis is often useful, but is not required if p values are reported (choice D can be eliminated).

Appendix
Some Lab Techniques

The material in this section is not *strictly* MCAT material; it is presented in this appendix as a reference source. In other words, you don't need to memorize it, but do read it for familiarity. The MCAT is a test of your ability to deal with new material like this, presented on the exam in passage form.

A.1 ENZYME-LINKED IMMUNO-SORBENT ASSAY (ELISA)

As the name suggests, an ELISA is a biochemical technique that utilizes antigen-antibody interactions ("immuno-sorbency") to determine the presence of either

- antigens (like proteins or cytokines), or
- specific immunoglobulins (antibodies)

in a sample (such as cells recovered from a tumor biopsy or a patient's serum). Figure 1 illustrates the basic protocol when testing for the presence of a specific antigen.

Step 1: The experimental wells are coated with antibodies that are specific for the target antigen.

Step 2: A sample of serum or cell extract is added to the wells.

Step 3: The antibodies immobilize the antigen by binding to it (if it is present in the sample).

Step 4: Any unbound proteins remaining in the sample are washed away.

Step 5: An enzyme-linked antibody that also recognizes the target protein is added to the wells.

Step 6: The wells are filled with a solution that changes color in the presence of the detection enzyme (the one linked to the antibody added in Step 5). A color change indicates the target protein was present in the sample; no color change means the protein was absent.

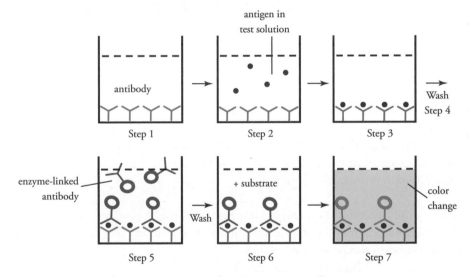

Figure 1   Testing for the Presence of Antigen

When testing for the presence of a specific antibody in a sample, the *antigen* (for which the antibody is specific) is first allowed to adhere directly to the wells. The sample is added as above, and then mixed with enzyme-linked antibodies (see Figure 2).

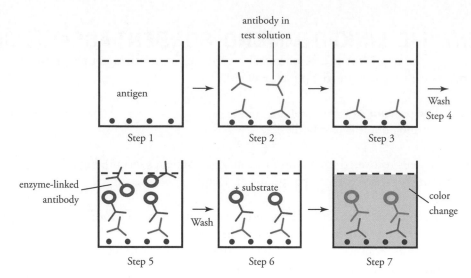

Figure 2   Testing for the Presence of Antibody

ELISA can be used to screen patients for viral infections. For example, serum from a patient suspected to be infected with HIV is loaded into wells that are coated with HIV coat proteins. If the serum contains anti-HIV antibodies (indicating infection), the antibodies will adhere to the proteins on the wells, bind enzyme-linked antibodies, and effect a color change.

A.2   RADIOIMMUNOASSAY (RIA)

RIAs are similar to ELISAs but use radiolabeled antibodies rather than enzyme-linked antibodies. Thus, the presence of target proteins or antibodies is assayed by measuring the amount of radioactivity instead of a color change. RIAs are more extensively used in the medical field to measure the relative amounts of hormones or drugs in patients' sera (see Figure 3).

Step 1: A known amount of radiolabeled antigen (for example, insulin that was synthesized with ^{125}I-labeled tyrosines) is incubated with a known amount of antibody that is specific to the antigen.

Step 2: The insulin:antibody complexes are isolated.

Step 3: The total amount of radioactivity is measured.

Step 4: Unlabeled insulin (also called *cold insulin*) is mixed into the solution in increasing amounts. The cold insulin competes with the labeled insulin (*hot insulin*) for the antibody. As more cold insulin is added, less total radioactivity is recovered and measured. This competition assay helps formulate a standard curve (see Figure 4).

Step 5: Steps 1–3 are repeated using patient serum instead of the cold insulin. The standard curve is used to extrapolate the amount of insulin that is circulating in a patient's serum.

Figure 3   Radioimmunoassay (RIA)

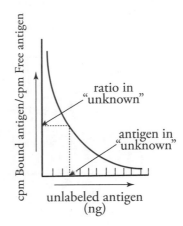

Figure 4   Standard Curve

A.3   ELECTROPHORESIS

Electrophoresis is a means of separating things by size (for example, nucleic acids or proteins) or by charge (for example, proteins or individual amino acids). A "gel" is made out of either acrylamide or agarose by solubilizing the acrylamide or agarose, pouring it into a rectangular mold, and then allowing it to cool and solidify. Acrylamide and agarose form "nets" as they solidify; the more acrylamide or agarose used in the initial solution, the smaller the pores in the nets.

The mold used to pour the gel creates wells in the gel into which samples can be loaded. An electrical current is applied such that the end of the gel with the wells is negatively charged and the opposite end is positively charged. This causes the samples to migrate toward the positive pole, according to size; smaller things migrate faster (because they fit more easily through the pores of the gel) and larger things migrate more slowly.

For example, here are the steps for separating DNA fragments by size.

Step 1:   Isolate the sample DNA from cells.

Step 2:   Expose the DNA to enzymes called **restriction endonucleases** (see Section A.5), which cleave the strands of DNA into smaller fragments of varying size. This may not be necessary in some cases.

Step 3:   Add a loading dye to the DNA sample. This makes the sample visible as it is being loaded into the gel. Loading dye also contains a chemical to help inhibit DNA degradation. Finally, glycerol in the loading dye makes the sample more dense than the surrounding buffer, which means the DNA sample sinks to the bottom of the gel wells.

Step 4: Load the mixture of fragments into the gel wells and apply the electrical current (this is called "running a gel"). Each strand of DNA (negatively charged!) migrates toward the positive end of the gel, but the smaller fragments migrate more quickly, so they are found farther from the wells at any point in the experiment. You run the samples alongside a "standard" lane, which contains fragments of known size (this helps identify the size of the unknowns).

Step 5: Visualize the bands of DNA in the gel. This is done using a dye that binds to nucleic acids and fluoresces when exposed to UV light. This dye is typically added to the gel when it is being made, but it can also be applied after the gel is run. The size of each DNA band can be approximated by comparing it to the ladder.

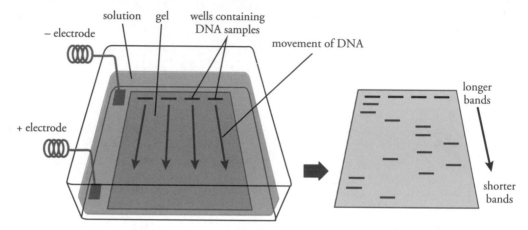

Figure 5   Agarose Gel Electrophoresis of DNA

In addition to determining their sizes, fragments of DNA (or RNA) in an electrophoresed gel can be transferred to a more solid and stable membrane in a process called "blotting." There are several types of blots used in biology laboratories.

A.4   BLOTTING

Simply put, blotting is the transfer of DNA or proteins from an electrophoresis gel to a nitrocellulose of PVDF membrane. Once transferred, further experiments can be run to isolate or detect a particular nucleic acid fragment or protein (called "probing"). Blotting is classified by the type of molecule being probed.

Southern Blotting

Southern blotting allows you detect the presence of specific sequences within a heterogeneous sample of DNA. This process also allows you to isolate and purify target sequences of DNA for further study.

Step 1: Separate the DNA fragments on an electrophoresis gel.

Step 2: Transfer the fragments to a nitrocellulose membrane.

Step 3: "Probe" the filter for the target DNA sequence. Hybridization probes are short single-stranded sequences of nucleic acid (usually DNA) that have two important features:

- They are complementary to (and thus will base-pair with) a portion of the target DNA sequence.
- They are constructed with radiolabeled nucleotides, which allows the visualization of the target sequence with special film.

Probes are often engineered to complement mutations or certain gene rearrangements, making Southern blotting a useful diagnostic tool.

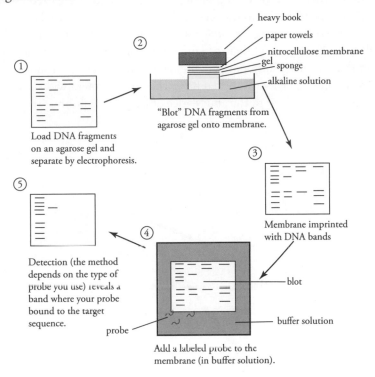

Figure 6   Southern Blotting

Northern Blotting

Northern blotting is almost identical to Southern blotting, except that RNA is separated via gel electrophoresis instead of DNA. The rest of the process is the same; once the RNA has been separated on a gel, it is transferred to a nitrocellulose membrane and detected via radiolabeled nucleic acid probe. This technique allows you to determine whether specific gene products (normal or pathologic) are being expressed (if their mRNA is present in a cell, they are probably being translated to protein).

Western Blotting

Western blotting allows you to detect the presence of certain proteins within a sample and also serves as a diagnostic tool. You are able to determine, for example, whether cancer cells express certain tumor-promoting growth receptors on their surface. Here are the steps.

Step 1: Cells are collected and solubilized in detergent to release their cytoplasmic contents.
Step 2: Cell lysates, which contain hundreds of different proteins, are denatured (meaning they lose their secondary and tertiary structures). Lysates and a ladder are loaded onto a gel. Similar to nucleic acid gel electrophoresis, a ladder is used so protein size can be compared to a standard.
Step 3: An electric current is applied. Because of the detergent used, the proteins are all negatively charged. Therefore, they migrate toward the positive electrode, with the smaller proteins migrating the farthest from the wells.
Step 4: The separated proteins from the gel are transferred to a nitrocellulose or PVDF membrane.

Step 5: The membrane is probed for the target protein. Probing for proteins in Western blotting differs from probing in Southern or Northern blotting in that antibodies are used as the probes rather than nucleic acids. This is similar to the technique in ELISA; a primary antibody is used first, which will recognize only the target protein via its antigen-binding portions. Then, an enzyme-linked secondary antibody is used that recognizes the constant region of the primary antibody. The enzyme on the secondary antibody will fluoresce when a detection substrate is added, and this light can be photographed with special film. The target protein will show up as a band with an intensity that is proportional to the abundance of the protein in the sample (see Figure 7).

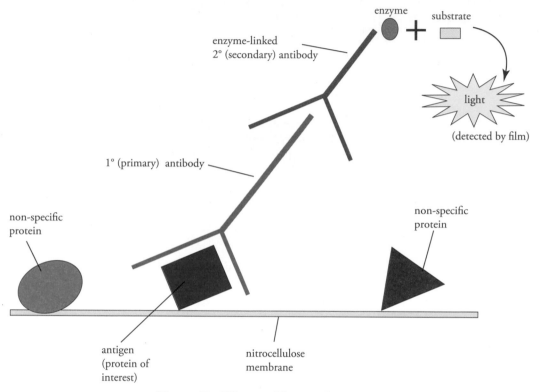

Figure 7   Western Blotting Detection

Eastern Blotting

Several variations of Eastern blotting have been reported, but these tests are not commonly used in molecular biology labs. Eastern blots are used to analyze post-translational modification of peptides, such as the addition of lipids or carbohydrates. The details of this protocol depend on the specifics of the experiment.

A.5 RECOMBINANT DNA

In the past 20 years, a major change has occurred in biology that has allowed it to not only describe the mechanisms of life, but also to manipulate living organisms. The cloning and sequencing of genes, production of recombinant DNA, and the subsequent production of recombinant proteins for use as therapeutic agents in medicine have now become commonplace procedures. A **recombinant protein** is one which has been obtained by transcribing and translating a novel combination of DNA (**recombinant DNA**) from different organisms. For example, the gene for human insulin can be placed in a bacterial **plasmid** (described below). Bacteria with the plasmid will then produce insulin that can be used to treat diabetes. To a large extent, these advances are due to the development of new technologies for the handling of DNA, such as the discovery of restriction endonucleases that cleave particular DNA sequences.

Restriction endonucleases are bacterial enzymes that recognize specific sequences of DNA and cut the double-stranded molecule in two pieces. A **nuclease** is an enzyme that cuts nucleic acids. An **endonuclease** cuts in the middle of a DNA chain (contrast with **exonucleases**, which nibble nucleotides from the ends of DNA chains). They are isolated from bacteria and used in the lab. Their natural role in the bacterium is to destroy viral DNA that gets injected into the cell; thus, they *restrict* the reproduction of hostile viruses.

Restriction enzymes have found great use in molecular biology, where they have permitted manipulation of genes to create recombinant DNA. For example, in Figure 8 below, the cutting-specificity of a restriction enzyme known as *Eco*RI is shown (other restriction enzymes cut at different sequences). The free ends of the DNA molecule that were complementary are known as **sticky ends** since they are able to base pair with other DNA molecules with similar sequences.

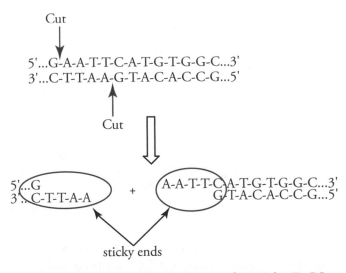

Figure 8   Restriction Digestion of DNA by *Eco*RI

Study the sequence shown in Figure 8. Notice anything in particular? If you read the top strand from left to right (5' to 3'), it begins GAATTC. Now read the bottom strand from right to left (still 5' to 3'), but only read the six nucleotides on the *left* side of the chain. It says GAATTC (same as above)! Just looking at these six nucleotides, we see that the chain possesses **two-fold rotational symmetry**. The six 5' nucleotides of the top chain are the same as the six 3' nucleotides of the bottom one. Sequences with two-fold rotational symmetry are known as **palindromes**. Many restriction enzymes recognize palindromic sequences.

When a fragment of double-stranded DNA is created by cutting with a restriction endonuclease, it can be inserted into DNA from any source that was also digested by the same restriction endonuclease. For example, *Eco*RI-generated DNA fragments from a human can be isolated, mixed with *Eco*RI-digested DNA from a bacterial plasmid, and then joined by the enzyme DNA ligase. Hybrid DNA produced in this fashion is referred to as recombinant DNA.

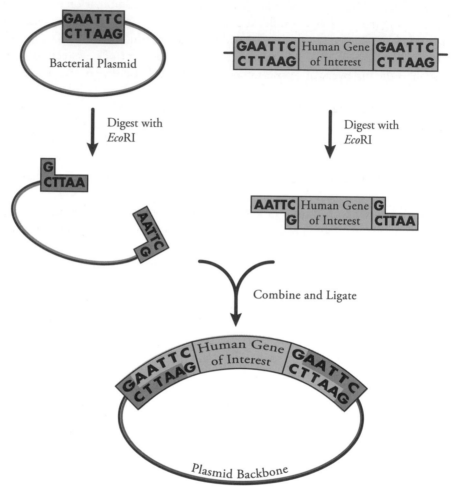

Figure 9   Cloning DNA Using a Sticky-End Restriction Enzyme

Some restriction enzymes generate DNA with blunt ends rather than sticky ends. That is, the 3' and 5' ends at the cut site are even, with no overhanging bases. Ligating blunt ends together is less specific, and restriction sites may or may not be retained. For example, if the same blunt-cutting restriction enzyme is used on both pieces of DNA, the restriction site will be maintained after ligation. If different blunt-cutting enzymes are used, the products can be ligated together but neither restriction site will be maintained. In Figure 10, a bacterial plasmid was digested with the restriction enzyme *Sma*I (which is a blunt cutter and recognizes the restriction site CCCGGG). A human gene of interest was digested with the restriction enzyme *Eco*RV (which is a blunt cutter and recognizes the sequence GATATC). Notice that both these restriction sites are six base pair palindromes. Because both enzymes generate blunt ends, these products can be ligated together. However, the recombinant DNA has lost the restriction sites for both enzymes. The DNA that remains is a combination of the two blunt sites (CCCATC and GATGGG), and it cannot be digested with either *Sma*I or *Eco*RV.

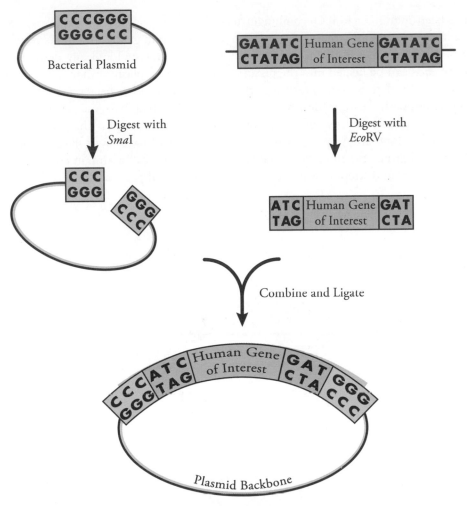

Figure 10   Cloning DNA Using Two Blunt-End Restriction Enzymes

Plasmids

Plasmids are small circular ds-DNA molecules found in bacteria that are capable of autonomous replication (replication that is independent of chromosome replication). Plasmid replication still requires an origin of replication (ORI), and this affects the copy number of the plasmid. Some plasmids have strong ORIs, leading to hundreds of plasmid copies per cell. Other ORIs are less efficient, leading to only a few copies of the plasmid per cell. In addition, plasmid segregation during binary fission is not regulated. For high copy plasmids, both daughter cells will most likely end up with copies of the plasmid. For lower copy plasmids, one daughter cell could get all copies of the plasmid, while the other daughter cell gets none. Plasmids used in laboratories are almost always high copy plasmids. The presence of a large number of copies is convenient, since it allows for isolation of a large amount of plasmid DNA with identical sequences.

Plasmids have been manipulated by recombinant techniques to propagate and express foreign genes in bacteria. In addition to an ORI, they also contain a multiple cloning site, which has restriction sites for dozens of restriction enzymes. This means the plasmid can be digested and any desired sequence with complementary ends can be ligated into the plasmid. Furthermore, plasmids have a drug resistance gene that helps select and isolate bacteria possessing the plasmid from other bacteria. For example, bacteria containing a plasmid with the ampicillin-resistance gene are able to grow in the presence of the antibiotic ampicillin (and are AmpR, or resistant), while bacteria that do not possess the plasmid will die in the presence of ampicillin (and are AmpS, or sensitive). By growing all bacteria in the presence of ampicillin, only those bacteria that possess and express the plasmid can grow and maintain colonies (see Figure 11). Tetracycline, penicillin, and streptomycin are other commonly used prokaryotic selection agents.

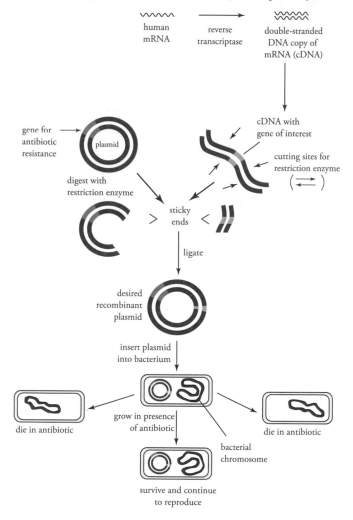

Figure 11   Expression of a Human Gene in Bacteria

Bacterial expression plasmids need extra components. A prokaryotic promoter and start site allow expression of an inserted gene in the bacterial host. The promoter can be either constitutively active or inducible upon addition of a chemical.

Bacterial Transformation

Plasmids can be easily reintroduced into bacterial cells via transformation. Transformation is a naturally occurring process, but only a very small percentage of bacteria are naturally willing to accept pieces of DNA floating around in their environment. These "competent" bacteria express special machinery that translocates the hydrophilic DNA across the lipid membrane. More often, the bacteria (or other cell types) must be coaxed to take up the plasmid. There are several ways to do this; the cells may be cooled in calcium chloride and then heat shocked to facilitate plasmid uptake. In another (called electroporation), an electric field is applied and this pokes holes in the membrane, which allows the plasmid to diffuse into the cell.

Once inside the bacteria, the plasmid will be exposed to the host's replication machinery, which replicates the plasmid (remember, it has its own origin of replication). If you are working with an expression plasmid, the DNA is also exposed to bacterial transcription machinery (remember, the plasmid contains the proper promoters and start signals). Newly synthesized mRNA can then access host ribosomes, which translate the encoded protein; on completion of translation, the cells are lysed to release the protein.

If the plasmid remains within the cytosol of the bacterium, the transformation is referred to as transient. In contrast, some plasmids are constructed to integrate within the host's genome. These stable transformations allow the plasmid to be replicated each time the bacterium replicates its own genome.

Complementary DNA

Many applications of DNA technology involve expressing eukaryotic genes in prokaryotic cells such as *E. coli*. This is conceptually simple: all you have to do is get eukaryotic DNA into a plasmid and get the plasmid into a bacterium, and the bacterium should express the gene. However, there are two main problems that need to be overcome. First, prokaryotes lack the equipment necessary for splicing out introns. Second, many eukaryotic genes are extremely long, making them hard to work with. One way to overcome these obstacles is to work with eukaryotic complementary DNA.

Complementary DNA (or cDNA) is produced from fully spliced eukaryotic mRNA. This is accomplished by a special enzyme you have encountered before: reverse transcriptase, obtained from retroviruses. This enzyme reads an RNA template and builds complementary DNA. Therefore, RNA can be isolated from a eukaryotic cell and converted into cDNA by the addition of reverse transcriptase, some generic primers and dNTP building blocks in buffer. cDNAs carry the complete coding sequences for genes, but they lack introns (and thus are smaller than the genomic sequence of the gene). Once a cDNA is ligated into a bacterial plasmid and bacteria are transformed with this plasmid, they can produce the protein encoded by the cDNA.

cDNA libraries are also commonly generated. This is where each of the thousands of mRNAs being generated by a given cell type or tissue are converted into cDNAs. Each cDNA is then cloned into a plasmid. This generates thousands of plasmids (the library), with each one containing one cDNA molecule. cDNA libraries can be compared across tissue types of a certain organism (brain versus liver, for example) to study tissue-specific gene expression.

Artificial Chromosomes

Plasmids can carry inserts only up to a certain size. If large inserts are required, artificial chromosomes can be used. Bacterial artificial chromosomes (BACs) typically carry inserts of 100 to 350 kilobase pairs (kb), while yeast artificial chromosomes (YACs) can carry inserts between 100 and 3,000 kb. In other words, BACs can easily carry up to 350,000 base pairs of DNA, and YACs can contain up to 3 million base pair inserts!

BACs contains sequences to allow replication and regulation of copy number, partition genes that promote their even distribution after bacterial cell division, and a selectable marker for antibiotic resistance. BACs that express inserted sequences also contain promoter regions.

YACs contain a centromere, telomeres, and sequences that function as replication origins. They also typically contain a gene that allows tryptophan or pyrimidine biosynthesis, allowing for selection of auxotrophic cells that contain the artificial chromosome. This system works similarly to antibiotic selection in bacteria.

BACs can be used to study inherited diseases that involve complex genes with several regulatory sequences and promoters upstream of the coding sequence. The entire gene can be cloned into a BAC, and this can be used to model genetic diseases in mice. For example, both Alzheimer's disease and Down syndrome have been studied in this way. BACs have also been used to clone the entire genome of some viruses, such as herpesviruses, poxviruses, and coronaviruses. These infective BACs initiate viral infection in the host cell and have facilitated research on these viruses.

Both BACs and YACs were initially used in the Human Genome Project, to help make chromosome maps. However, YACs were eventually abandoned because they are less stable than BACs. Despite this, they do have one major advantage: because yeast cells are eukaryotic, YACs can be used to express and study proteins that require post-translational modification.

Eukaryotic Plasmids

Eukaryotic plasmids also exist. They require many of the same components as bacterial plasmids. Eukaryotes use different selection agents, usually either puromycin or neomycin. They also require different promoters in expression plasmids, as well as a poly-adenylation signal downstream of the inserted gene, to terminate transcription.

Eukaryotic plasmids can be introduced into mammalian host cells via transfection. Similar to transformation, there are several experimental options for transfection. Cells can be chemically transfected, usually using calcium phosphate precipitates or plasmid packaging in liposomes. These lipid vesicles mask the plasmid, but they deliver it to the interior of the cell by fusing with the plasma membrane. Non-chemical options for transfection include electroporation, optical transfection with lasers, or shooting the DNA coupled to a gold nanoparticle into a cell nucleus using a gene gun.

Viruses can also deliver DNA into eukaryotic cells, a process called viral transduction. Transduced cells can express genes carried by the viral vector.

A.6 POLYMERASE CHAIN REACTION

Polymerase chain reaction (PCR) is a very quick and inexpensive method for detecting and amplifying specific DNA sequences, screening hereditary and infectious diseases, cloning genes, and fingerprinting DNA. Designed to generate myriad copies of a single template sequence, PCR allows the amplification and subsequent analysis of very small samples of DNA.

Let's say that PCR is to be used to determine whether a certain viral gene has been integrated within a bacterial host genome. A nuclear extract of the bacteria is obtained. Then primers are carefully constructed that will help locate the viral gene (if it is present within the host). Primers are engineered DNA oligonucleotides (~15 bases of single stranded DNA) that will recognize and base pair with specific DNA sequences; in this example, the primers will each recognize a 15-base stretch of the viral gene. Two primers, which will flank a total of ~10 kb of DNA, are used. The "forward primer" will recognize a 15-base stretch at the 3' end of the antisense strand, and the "reverse primer" will recognize a 15-base stretch at the 3' end of the sense strand. When base-paired to their respective gene sequences, the primers will bookend (on opposite sides) the intervening target gene segment (see Figure 12).

Figure 12   PCR Primers

The primers have free 3' hydroxyl groups to which dNTPs can be added in a 5' to 3' direction. This will allow the elongation of complementary strands of DNA. The bacterial DNA is mixed with multiple copies of the forward and reverse primers, lots of dNTP bases, a heat-sensitive DNA polymerase, and ions into a buffer. The mixture is then placed into a PCR machine, which will carry out three basic steps (see Figure 13):

Step 1: <u>Initialization</u>. The sample is heated to ~95°C. Heating the sample "melts" the hydrogen bonds that hold the ds-DNA together, which creates single-stranded DNA.

Step 2: <u>Annealing</u>. The sample is cooled to ~55°C. At this temperature, the primers base-pair with the template strands.

Step 3: <u>Elongation</u>. The sample is heated to ~72°C. Using the primers as starting points, the heat-sensitive DNA polymerase (usually *Taq* polymerase isolated from algae that thrive in hot springs) elongates strands of DNA that are complementary to each of the template strands. Each strand is polymerized in the 5' to 3' direction. Any mismatched primers will dissociate from the template strands and will not be extended (this helps ensure the purity of the PCR product). Longer DNA targets take longer to synthesize, so the length of the elongation step depends on the length of the product DNA.

A.6

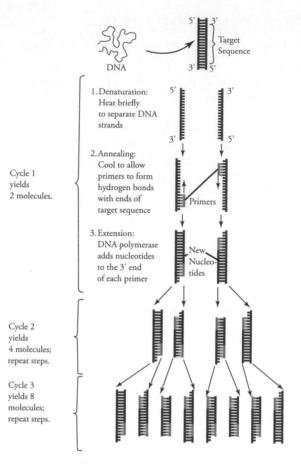

Figure 13   PCR Steps

Each cycle of three steps takes between 0.5 and 5 minutes, depending on the length of the target DNA product (and subsequent length of the elongation step). Because two new complementary strands are synthesized for each template strand in the sample, the PCR product grows at an exponential rate, yielding over a billion copies in just 30 cycles. The sample of DNA is separated via electrophoresis and stained to visualize the products, including the amplified viral gene segment (if present).

Reverse Transcriptase-Polymerase Chain Reaction (RT-PCR)

This is an extension of classic PCR and is used to detect the relative expression of specific gene products. While RT-PCR does not measure the actual expression or abundance of proteins, the technique provides a gauge of gene transcription by measuring the relative amount of target mRNAs. To conduct an RT-PCR experiment, all of the mRNAs from within a cell population are first isolated and then converted into complementary DNA (cDNA) using the enzyme reverse transcriptase. This "library" of cDNAs is then subjected to PCR, using primers specific for a certain gene of interest. If the gene was actively transcribed at the time of harvest, its mRNA will have yielded a cDNA, which will be amplified by the PCR reaction and visualized on a gel.

Quantitative Polymerase Chain Reaction (qPCR)

In quantitative PCR (qPCR, also called real-time PCR), the PCR product is both detected and quantified, either as an absolute number of copies or as a relative amount normalized to a control. The amplified DNA is detected in "real time," as the reaction progresses. The detection process can either use a dye that is fluorescent and binds DNA or a fluorescent oligonucleotide probe which hybridizes to the sequence of interest. qPCR can be performed on either DNA or cDNA templates, meaning it can give information on the presence and abundance of a particular DNA sequence in samples (if DNA is the template) or on gene expression (if the template is cDNA).

A.7 DNA SEQUENCING AND GENOMICS

DNA sequencing is a method by which scientists can determine gene sequences. This provides the basis for investigating the genetics of health and disease. Knowing gene sequences is also a critical component of other experimental techniques, for example, when constructing primers for PCR reactions.

The most widely used DNA sequencing method (the Sanger technique) hinges on a simple yet important structural characteristic of DNA molecules. The ringed ribose of a dNTP has various substituents attached to its carbons: a nitrogenous base at the 1' carbon, a hydrogen at the 2' carbon (recall that a hydroxyl group occupies this site in RNA), a hydroxyl group at the 3' carbon, and a string of three phosphates at the 5' carbon. The 3' carbon hydroxyl group serves as the binding site for another dNTP. Without a free 3' carbon hydroxyl group, dNTPs could not be linked together, and DNA synthesis would not be possible. The Sanger technique utilizes a modified dNTP, which lacks the 3' carbon hydroxyl group. These dideoxynucleotide triphosphates (ddNTPs) maintain their 5' carbon triphosphate moiety and can be incorporated normally into a growing DNA molecule; however, because they are lacking the 3' carbon hydroxyl group, no further bases can be added to them. Thus, these ddNTPs terminate stand elongation at the point of their insertion. The basic protocol is as follows (see Figure 14):

Step 1: Obtain a sample of DNA to sequence.

Step 2: Denature the DNA into single strands.

Step 3: Mix the sample of DNA with radiolabeled primers, DNA polymerase, and a mixture of dCTP, dTTP, dGTP, dATP, and ddATP (with the dideoxy form making up 1 percent of the adenine base population). This step of the assay will yield a population of newly synthesized DNA fragments, varying in length, each complimentary to the template strand and covalently bonded to a radiolabeled primer at the 5' end (this will aid in the detection of the newly synthesized fragments later). The variety in length of the fragments results from the random insertion of a ddATP into the growing chain.

Step 4: Conduct three more separate reactions as in the previous step, using each of the three other bases in dideoxy form (ddCTP, ddGTP, and ddTTP).

Step 5: Separate the fragments via gel electrophoresis, running each reaction from Steps 3 and 4 in a separate lane.

Step 6: Transfer the fragments to a membrane and visualize them with radio-sensitive film.

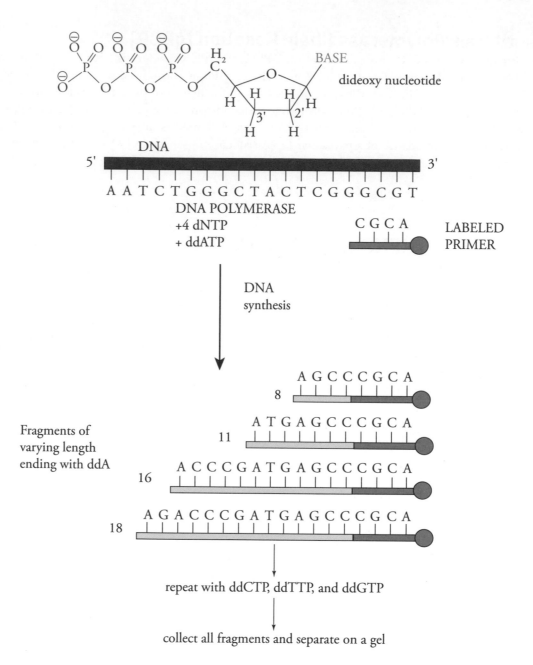

Figure 14 DNA Sequencing Reactions

The smallest fragment (i.e., the fragment that migrates the farthest from the well) is a primer with only a single ddNTP attached to it. The lane it ran in corresponds to the first base incorporated into the strand which is the first base of the sequence of the complimentary strand. The second smallest fragment is a primer with two bases attached; this fragment ran in the lane corresponding to the base at the second position in the complimentary strand (see Figure 15). Reading the membrane from bottom (farthest from the wells) to top (closest to the wells) indicates the sequence (in the 5' to 3' direction) of the complimentary strand. Remembering the simple rules of base-pairing (A:T and C:G), you can easily extrapolate the sequence of the template strand.

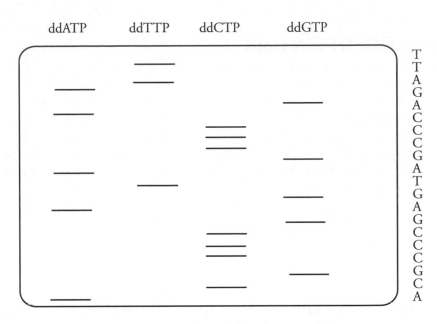

DNA sequence can be read from bottom of gel up

Figure 15 DNA Sequencing Gel

Genomics

The genome of the bacterium *Haemophilus influenzae* was the first to be sequenced and published in 1995. Since then, the genomes of hundreds of organisms have been sequenced and published, including humans and model organisms commonly used in biology laboratories (e.g., *E. coli*, *D. melanogaster*, etc.). Researchers and clinicians have recently started sequencing the genome of many cancers, which allows comparative studies between different types and subtypes of cancer, as well as a better understanding of how the cancer genome is different from a normal one.

Genomic sequencing is generally done in two ways, which can be complementary. The first strategy is to generate a genetic linkage map, with several hundred markers per chromosome. This map is then refined to a physical map by preparing YAC or BAC libraries containing large chromosomal fragments. The library is put in order and then gradually cloned into libraries containing smaller and smaller fragments. Each of these small fragments is eventually sequenced and assembled into an overall sequence.

The second strategy is a whole-genome shotgun approach, in which chromosomes are cut into small fragments, which are cloned and sequenced. This strategy skips generating maps, and because of this, requires much more extensive analysis of sequencing data by computers in order to align fragments.

Genomic data can lead to predictions on how many genes there are in a certain organism, where they are located, how expression is controlled, and how the genome is organized. It also supports larger questions, like how evolution and speciation occur. Finally, genomic data can be used to study genetic variation within and across species. Tools for analysis of genomic data have been developed and are always being refined. Researchers can now submit several different gene or protein sequences and receive a report that predicts how related the sequences are from an evolutionary point of view. There are also tools to align multiple sequences so we can study how similar and different they are.

A.8 DNA FINGERPRINTING

Much like visualizing subtle differences in the whorl pattern of a thumbprint, DNA fingerprinting allows scientists (and police departments!) to detect sequence variations that make each individual's DNA unique. The ability to appreciate subtle differences within different individuals' DNA comes in handy when matching a DNA sample from a murder suspect to the DNA in a drop of blood found at a crime scene, or when screening for disease-causing genes, or when doing paternity testing. Since the DNA of any two people is more than 99 percent identical, DNA fingerprinting exploits stretches of repetitive and highly variable DNA called **polymorphisms**. These intervening 2–100 base-pair sequences of DNA are structurally variable with respect to their sequence, length, multiplicity, and location within the genome. Two of the several methods of fingerprinting are described below, **restriction fragment length polymorphism** (RFLP) analysis and **short tandem repeat** (STR) analysis.

A.8

Restriction Fragment Length Polymorphism (RFLP) Analysis

Step 1: This method uses restriction endonucleases to cut 10–100 base-pair stretches of polymorphic DNA (called minisatellites) into small fragments. Because of the size variations inherent in this DNA, the resulting DNA fragments (now referred to as RFLPs) also vary in size and are unique to an individual.

Step 2: The RFLPs are separated via gel electrophoresis and transferred to a membrane. Southern blotting techniques are used to analyze the sample. The membrane is probed with radiolabeled DNA oligonucleotides that base-pair with specific RFLP sequences, and the membrane is visualized with special film. Polymorphic DNA, even though recovered from the same chromosomal region, will yield unique band distributions for each person. When RFLPs are recovered from DNA sequences within genes, mutations can be detected. For example, sickle cell disease is caused by a single base substitution in the beta chain of hemoglobin. The substituted valine at the sixth position (normally, glutamic acid is present) will introduce a novel restriction site within the gene. When cut with restriction endonucleases, the point mutation generates a different sized RFLP (when compared to the normal gene cut with the same enzymes) and will yield an anomalous banding pattern (see Figure 16).

Short Tandem Repeat (STR) Analysis

Step 1: This method uses PCR to amplify 5–10 base-pair stretches of highly polymorphic and repetitive DNA located within noncoding (introns) regions of the genome. These STRs vary with respect to the sequence and number of repeats found at each locus. To profile an individual, a sample of DNA is obtained and the polymorphic DNA is amplified with PCR.

Step 2: The amplified STRs are separated via electrophoresis and analyzed with Southern blotting.

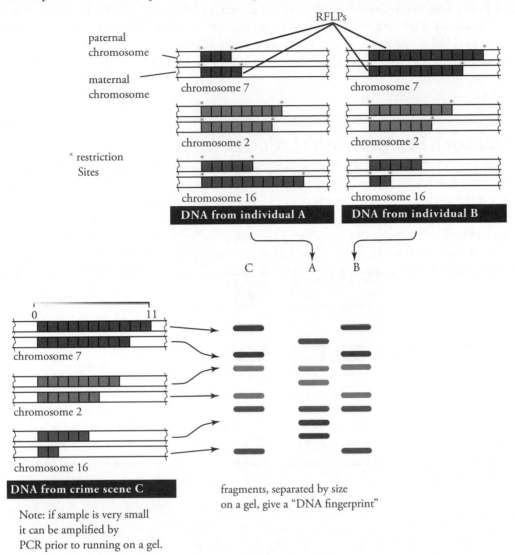

Figure 16 RFLP Analysis

A.9 ADDITIONAL METHODS TO STUDY THE GENOME

Genomic sequencing is the ultimate study of the genome. However, it is very costly and takes a long time. Depending on the experiment, one of the following methods may be better suited to answering a biological question.

Exome and Targeted Sequencing

Instead of sequencing the entire genome, scientists can target only certain regions of interest. Exome sequencing involves sequencing only the exons of the genome. On a smaller scale, individual genes can be sequenced. These selective techniques involve enriching the DNA of interest (by amplification for example), followed by standard sequencing.

A.9

Karyotyping

When generating a karyotype, scientists order all the chromosomes from 1 to 22 plus the sex chromosomes, for a genome-wide view of genetic information. Chromosomes are stained (using Giemsa stain) to highlight structural features. Major genetic changes (involving millions of base pairs), aneuploidy (when a cell contains an abnormal number of chromosomes), and some insertions, deletions, or translocations can be revealed.

Fluorescence *in situ* Hybridization

Fluorescence *in situ* hybridization (FISH) uses fluorescently labeled probes to locate the positions of specific DNA sequences on chromosomes. This detects and localizes the presence or absence of specific DNA sequences on chromosomes. Fluorescence microscopy is used to find out where the fluorescent probe is bound to the chromosomes. For example, large chromosomal translocations have been found in several types of cancer. A translocation between chromosomes 2 and 3 is often found in follicular thyroid carcinoma. This translocation produces a fusion gene that contains the promoter from one gene and the coding sequence of another. FISH analysis using chromosome 2 and 3 probes can detect and diagnose this translocation.

A.10   ANALYZING GENE EXPRESSION

Many of the techniques discussed above give information about gene expression. For example, RT-PCR and qPCR give information on which genes are being transcribed in a given cell population. Western blot analysis can directly test protein expression, and it is limited only by the amount of starting lysate and the availability of antibodies specific for the protein being studied. Additional methods have been developed to study gene expression. Each of these techniques can be used to study a certain gene and gather information about its expression and function, or they can be used to study certain cells and gain information on which genes they are expressing and how they grow and survive.

Microarrays

Microarrays can be used to study relative RNA amounts between two samples or to compare RNA levels in one sample to a normal reference. The two samples of RNA (either two different experimental samples being compared to each other, or one sample and a control) are reverse-transcribed into cDNA and labeled with fluorescent dyes of different colors, then mixed and applied to an array chip. This chip contains binding sites for every known gene, which act as probes to determine transcript levels in the samples. For example, in Figure 17, gene expression is being compared between two tissue samples (A and B) using a hybridization microarray. The cDNA generated from sample A is labeled red, and cDNA generated from sample B is labeled green. Samples are mixed and applied to the chip. Genes 1 and 5 are more highly expressed in Sample A, since these sites on the chip are red. Genes 2 and 4 are more highly expressed in Sample B, since these sites on the chip are green. Gene 3 is expressed in both samples in approximately equal amount resulting in yellow. Microarray data is quantitative, and actual fold-changes can be calculated based on color and intensity.

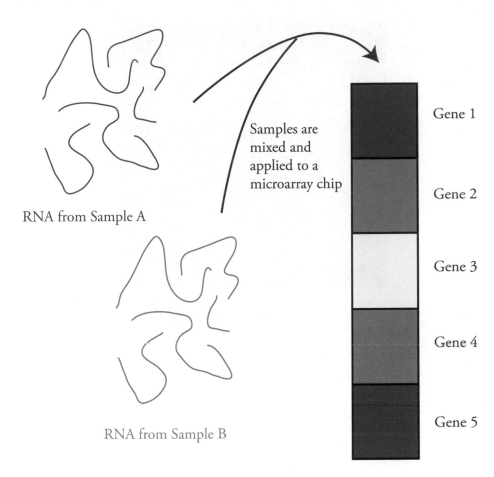

Figure 17 Transcriptional Profiling via Microarray

In situ Hybridization

In situ hybridization (ISH) can be used to determine expression of a gene of interest in a tissue, or in an embryo. A very thin slice (or "section") of a tissue sample is mounted onto a microscope slide. The tissue is fixed to keep transcripts in place, and then it is permeabilized to open the cell membrane. A labeled probe, which is specific for the transcript of interest, is added to the section and binds to the transcript being studied. An enzyme-linked antibody is added and binds to the probe. When a substrate for the enzyme is added, the target transcript-probe-antibody complex is detected. In this way, it can be determined when and where transcripts are expressed on a multicellular level.

Immunohistochemistry

This technique is similar to ISH, but it is specific for proteins instead of nucleic acids. As such, it gives a direct report on protein expression in a tissue. Immunohistochemistry (IHC) requires an antibody against a known protein. This antibody is recognized by a secondary antibody, which is either linked to an enzyme or a fluorescent molecule. IHC is commonly used in the clinic. For example, breast cancer biopsies from women are stained for the estrogen receptor (ER), the progesterone receptor (PR), and a plasma membrane receptor called HER2. Breast tumors are then classified as ER⁺ or ER⁻, PR⁺ or PR⁻, and HER2⁺ or HER2⁻. These classifications affect which therapy the patient is given.

Figure 18 Using Immunofluorescence to Determine Subcellular Protein Expression

In Figure 18, cells were stained with three different markers: the plasma membrane was labeled in green, the nucleus was labeled in blue, and the protein of interest was labeled in red. Four different staining patterns are observed. The two cells at the top express the protein of interest in the cytoplasm. The three cells in the middle do not express the protein of interest. The cell on the bottom left expresses the protein of interest in the nucleus; the blue nuclear stain and red protein of interest stain are overlapping to make the nucleus purple. In the bottom right cell, the protein of interest is expressed on the plasma membrane. Co-expression of the green plasma membrane marker and the red protein of interest cause yellow staining of the plasma membrane.

Flow Cytometry

Flow cytometry again uses many of the same principles already discussed. Here, single cells (either from lab cultures or tissue samples) are stained for certain protein markers using specific antibodies. The antibodies are then linked to a fluorescent tag. Next, the labeled cells are suspended in a fluid stream and passed through a beam of light. Light detectors are found on the other side of, and perpendicular to, the laser. As the labeled cells pass through the light, the beam scatters and the fluorescent tag(s) on the cells can emit light. This combination of scattered and emitted light is measured to give information on cell size and how many cells in the sample express each of the markers that were labeled. Flow cytometers can have over a dozen different light channels, so many labeled antibodies can be added to one experimental sample. In addition to being analyzed, cells can also be sorted as they go through the machine (a technique called fluorescence-activated cell sorting, or FACS). In this way, a heterogeneous mixture of cells can be sorted based on expression of markers.

For example, the earliest (or least differentiated) thymocytes in the thymus express neither CD4 nor CD8; therefore, they are classed as double-negative (CD4$^-$CD8$^-$) cells. As these cells progress through their development, they become double-positive thymocytes (CD4$^+$CD8$^+$), and they finally mature to single-positive (CD4$^+$CD8$^-$ helper T-cells, or CD4$^-$CD8$^+$ killer T-cells) thymocytes that are then released from the thymus to peripheral tissues. Each of these four cell populations could be studied using flow cytometry (to determine their relative amounts for example) and could be isolated from each other using FACS.

A.11 PROTEIN QUANTIFICATION

A good understanding of genomics has led to the field of **proteomics**, the systematic and large-scale study of protein structure and function. This is usually done in a particular context, such as in a certain biochemical pathway, organelle, cell, tissue, or organism. Often, this involves quantitative analysis of proteins. This means measuring amounts of different proteins from a functional standpoint, looking at how the amount, state, or location of a protein changes. Here are some examples.

- It's been hypothesized that a particular protein under study functions in G_1 of the cell cycle, but not the other phases. A biochemist tags the protein with a fluorescent molecule, and observes live and cycling cells under a fluorescent microscope. He finds that the cells have high levels of fluorescence in G_1, but very low levels of fluorescence in the other cell phases. This suggests the protein under study is expressed at high levels in G_1 and then is degraded at the beginning of S phase.

- A biochemist is studying the function of an unknown protein, which has been shown to have important functions when a specific transcription factor is mutated. The biochemist obtains two cell lines. One has a mutation in the transcription factor, and the other doesn't. She generates lysate samples from the two cell lines. [This means she collects and lyses cells, releasing cellular proteins. Other macromolecules (such as lipid bilayers, DNA and RNA) are cleared or degraded by enzymes.] She then examines the two lysate samples, looking specifically at the protein of interest. She finds it is not phosphorylated in the cell line without the transcription factor mutation, but is phosphorylated in the cell line with the mutation.

- A biochemist has a culture of actively growing cells and applies a drug that is being tested for its therapeutic use. The drug targets a protein normally found in the nucleus of the cell. Addition of the drug causes the protein to be transported out of the nucleus and into the cytoplasm. A quantitative protein experiment measured the total amount of protein in different parts of the cell before and after treatment. It found 90% of the protein in the nucleus before drug treatment, and only 15% was in the nucleus after drug treatment.

Many different techniques can help with studying proteins quantitatively. Some of these look at proteins in a cell, either alive (FACS, labeling a protein and looking and subcellular location) or not (immunohistochemistry, flow cytometry). Others measure proteins harvested from a cell (ELISA, Western blotting, immunoprecipitation). All of these techniques are discussed earlier in this in Appendix.

It's common for proteins to be grown in a biological system and then extracted and studied. Often, protein levels in lysates or purified samples must be quantified before an experiment can be started. For example, before performing a Western blot, biochemists typically measure protein concentrations in each sample being studied, to make sure the same amount of lysate is loaded into each well of the gel.

A.11

The most commonly used quantification method is Bradford Quantification, using UV-Vis spectrophotometers designed for biochemical analysis. This method uses a Bradford reagent containing a blue pigment called Coomassie blue. When proteins bind the pigment, it shifts the absorption peak of the sample (Figure 19). Absorption is measured at 600 nm. This technique is very simple and has good sensitivity.

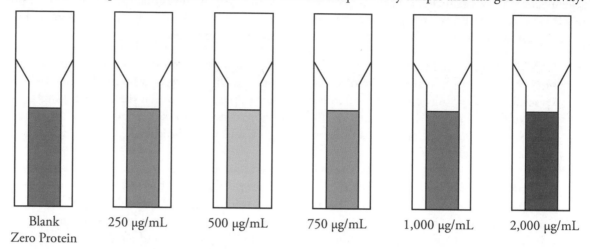

| Blank Zero Protein | 250 µg/mL | 500 µg/mL | 750 µg/mL | 1,000 µg/mL | 2,000 µg/mL |

Figure 19 Bradford Quantification of Proteins

To perform quantification, first, the negative control sample is put in the spectrophotometer, to set the zero value. Next, the samples with known concentration are applied, and the spectrophotometer generates a concentration curve. This relates absorbance of the sample with protein concentration. A new curve should be made every time proteins are being quantified. Next, the samples are put in the machine one by one. The spectrophotometer applies light in the visible and adjacent (near-UV and near-infrared) ranges. Absorbance is determined and compared to the calibration curve, and the machine usually reports both the absorbance and the subsequent protein concentration.

A.12

A.12 AFFINITY CHROMATOGRAPHY

Affinity chromatography, which is used to separate biochemical mixtures, is based on highly specific interactions between macromolecules. While affinity chromatography is most commonly used to purify proteins, it can also be used on other macromolecules (such as nucleic acids). It uses many of the same principles described above: you start with a heterogeneous mixture of molecules (such as cell lysate, growth media or blood). To isolate a protein of interest, you can either use an antibody or tag the protein with an affinity tag. (For example, His-tagged proteins can be purified with nickel-based resins and slightly basic conditions; the bound proteins are eluted by adding imidazole or by lowering the pH.) The target molecule is trapped on a stationary phase due to specific binding, and the stationary phase is washed to increase purity. The target protein is then released (or eluted) off the solid phase, in a highly purified state.

Biochemistry Glossary

After each definition, the section number in *MCAT Biochemistry Review* where the term is discussed is given.

acetyl-CoA

The first substrate in the Krebs cycle, produced primarily from the oxidation of pyruvate by the pyruvate dehydrogenase complex; however acetyl-CoA is also produced during fatty acid oxidation and protein catabolism. [**Section 5.3**]

activation energy (E_a)

The amount of energy required to produce the transition state of a chemical reaction. If the activation energy for a reaction is very high, the reaction occurs very slowly. Enzymes (and other catalysts) increase reaction rates by reducing activation energy. [**Section 3.2**]

active site

The three-dimensional site on an enzyme where substrates (reactants) bind and a chemical reaction is facilitated. [**Section 4.5**]

active site model

Also called the "lock and key" model, this states that the active site of an enzyme and its substrate are perfectly complementary. [**Section 4.5**]

adenine

One of the four aromatic bases found in DNA and RNA; also a component of ATP, NADH, and $FADH_2$. Adenine is a purine; it pairs with thymine (in DNA) and with uracil (in RNA). [**Section 7.2**]

allosteric regulation

The modification of enzyme activity through interaction of molecules with specific sites on the enzyme other than the active site (called allosteric sites). [**Section 4.6**]

amino acids

The building blocks (monomers) of proteins. There are 20 different amino acids. [**Section 4.1**]

amphoteric substance

A substance that can act as either an acid or a base; e.g., the conjugate base of a weak polyprotic acid. [**Section 3.4**]

anabolism

The process of building complex structures out of simpler precursors (for example, synthesizing proteins from amino acids). [**Section 3.3**]

antiparallel orientation

The normal configuration of double-stranded DNA in which the 5' end of one strand is paired with the 3' end of the other. [**Section 7.2**]

ATP synthase

A protein complex found in the inner membrane of the mitochondria. It is essentially a channel that allows H^+ ions to flow from the intermembrane space to the matrix (down the gradient produced by the enzyme complexes of the electron transport chain); as the H^+ ions flow through the channel, ATP is synthesized from ADP and P_i. [**Section 5.3**]

blotting

The transfer of DNA or proteins from an electrophoresis gel to a nitrocellulose filter. [**Section A.4**]

Brønsted-Lowry acid/base

Brønsted-Lowry acids are proton donors; Brønsted-Lowry bases are proton acceptors. [**Section 3.4**]

buffer solution

A solution that resists changes in pH when acids or bases are added; it is usually made up of a weak acid and its conjugate base. [**Section 3.4**]

catabolism

The process of breaking down large molecules into smaller precursors (e.g. digestion of starch into glucose). [**Section 3.3**]

catalyst

Something that increases the rate of a chemical reaction by reducing the activation energy for that reaction. The ΔG of the reaction remains unchanged. [**Section 3.2**]

centromere

A structure near the middle of eukaryotic chromosomes to which the fibers of the mitotic spindle attach during cell division. [**Section 7.2**]

cholesterol

A large, ring-shaped lipid found in cell membranes. Cholesterol is the precursor for steroid hormones and is used to manufacture bile salts. [**Sections 3.4 and 7.3**]

chromatin

DNA that is densely packed around histone proteins. The genes in heterochromatin are generally inaccessible to enzymes and are turned off. [**Section 7.2**]

chromosome

A single piece of double-stranded DNA; part of the genome of an organism. Prokaryotes have circular chromosomes, and eukaryotes have linear chromosomes. [**Section 7.2**]

citric acid cycle

See "Krebs cycle." [**Section 5.3**]

coenzyme

An organic molecule that associates non-covalently with an enzyme; it is required for the proper functioning of the enzyme. [**Section 4.6**]

coenzyme Q (ubiquinone)

A small non-protein electron carrier in the electron transport chain. [**Section 5.3**]

cofactor

An inorganic molecule that associates non-covalently with an enzyme; it is required for the proper functioning of the enzyme. [**Section 4.6**]

competitive inhibitor

An enzyme inhibitor that competes with substrate for binding at the active site of the enzyme. When the inhibitor is bound, no product can be made. [**Section 4.8**]

cooperativity

A type of substrate binding to a multi-active site enzyme, in which the binding of one substrate molecule modulates the binding of subsequent substrate molecules. If the substrate affinity of the other subunits increases, it is positive cooperativity. If the substrate affinity of the other subunits decreases, it is negative cooperativity. A graph of reaction rate vs. substrate concentration appears sigmoidal. Note that cooperativity can be found in other situations as well; for example, hemoglobin binds oxygen with positive cooperativity. [**Section 4.7**]

cristae

The folds of the inner membrane of a mitochondrion. [**Section 5.3**]

cytochrome C

A small, iron-containing protein in the electron transport chain. [**Section 5.3**]

cytosine

One of the four aromatic bases found in DNA and RNA. Cytosine is a pyrimidine; it pairs with guanine. [**Section 7.2**]

denaturation

To lose three-dimensional structure, as when a protein is exposed to high temperatures. [**Section 4.3**]

disaccharide

A molecule formed by joining two monosaccharides. Common disaccharides are maltose, sucrose, and lactose. [**Section 5.1**]

disulfide bridge

A covalent sulfur-sulfur bond between the side chains of two cysteine residues; it can be in the same peptide or between two different peptides. [**Section 4.3**]

electron transport chain

A series of enzyme complexes found along the inner mitochondrial membrane. NADH and $FADH_2$ are oxidized by these enzymes; the electrons are shuttled down the chain and are ultimately passed to oxygen to produce water. The electron energy is used to pump H^+ out of the mitochondrial matrix; the resulting H^+ gradient is subsequently used to drive the production of ATP. [**Section 5.3**]

electrophoresis

A means of separating things by size (for example, nucleic acids or proteins) or by charge (for example, proteins). [**Section A.3**]

ELISA

A biochemical technique that utilizes antigen-antibody interactions to determine the presence of either antigens (such as proteins or cytokines), or specific immunoglobulins (antibodies) in a sample (such as cells recovered from a tumor biopsy or a patient's serum). [**Section A.1**]

enzyme

A physiological catalyst. Enzymes are usually proteins, although some RNAs have catalytic activity. [**Sections 3.2 and 4.4**]

euchromatin

DNA that is loosely packed around histones. This DNA is more accessible to enzymes, and the genes in euchromatin can be activated if needed. [**Section 7.2**]

$FADH_2$

The reduced form (carries electrons) of FAD (flavin adenine dinucleotide). This is the other main electron carrier in cellular respiration (NADH is the most common). [**Section 5.3**]

fatty acid

A long chain hydrocarbon with a carboxylic acid functional group. [**Section 6.1**]

fatty acid oxidation

Also called beta-oxidation; the breakdown of fatty acids into acetyl-CoA molecules. [**Section 6.6**]

fatty acid synthase

The enzyme that synthesizes fatty acids from 2-carbon units derived from malonyl-CoA. This enzyme requires the reducing power of NADPH, obtained from the pentose phosphate pathway. [**Section 6.6**]

feedback inhibition
Also called *negative feedback*, the inhibition of an early step in a series of events by the product of a later step in the series. This has the effect of stopping the series of events when the products are plentiful and the series is unnecessary. Feedback inhibition is the most common form of regulation in the body, controlling such things as enzyme reactions, hormone levels, blood pressure, body temperature, and so on. [**Section 4.6**]

fermentation
The reduction of pyruvate to either ethanol or lactate in order to regenerate NAD⁺ from NADH. Fermentation occurs in the absence of oxygen and allows glycolysis to continue under those conditions. [**Section 5.3**]

flavoproteins
A protein associated with FAD that is commonly involved in redox reactions. [**Section 5.3**]

fructose-1,6-bisphosphatase
Dephosphorylates fru-1,6-bisP in gluconeogenesis. [**Section 5.5**]

futile cycling
The simultaneous activation of metabolic pathways with opposing roles, e.g., running glycolysis and gluconeogenesis at the same time. The tight regulation of metabolic pathways exists to prevent futile cycling. [**Section 5.5**]

gene
A portion of DNA that codes for some product, usually a protein, including all regulatory sequences. Some genes code for rRNA and tRNA, which are not translated. [**Section 7.2**]

genome
All the genetic information in an organism; all of an organism's chromosomes. [**Section 7.2**]

Gibbs free energy
The energy in a system that can be used to drive chemical reactions. If the change in free energy of a reaction (ΔG, the free energy of the products minus the free energy of the reactants) is negative, the reaction will occur spontaneously. [**Section 3.1**]

glucagon
A peptide hormone produced and secreted by the α cells of the pancreas. It targets primarily the liver, stimulating the breakdown of glycogen, thus increasing blood glucose levels. [**Section 5.5**]

gluconeogenesis
A metabolic pathway that synthesizes glucose from non-carbohydrate precursors. It occurs in the liver when dietary stores of glucose are unavailable and the liver has depleted its stores of glycogen and glucose. [**Section 5.4**]

glucose-6-phosphate dehydrogenase (G6PDH)
The enzyme that catalyzes the first step in the oxidative phase of the pentose phosphate pathway; it decarboxylates glucose-6-P to form ribulose-5-P and forms NADPH in the process. [**Section 5.7**]

glucose-6-phosphatase
The enzyme that decarboxylates glu-6-P in gluconeogenesis. This step is important so that glucose can exit the liver cell and enter the bloodstream. [**Section 5.5**]

glycogen phosphorylase
The enzyme that catalyzes the phosphorylation and subsequent removal of one glucose monomer at the end of a glycogen polymer. [**Sections 4.4 and 5.6**]

glycogen synthase
The enzyme that catalyzes the addition of glucose monomers to the glycogen polymer. [**Section 5.6**]

glycogenolysis
A term for glycogen breakdown. [**Section 5.6**]

glycolysis
The anaerobic splitting of a glucose molecule into 2 pyruvic acid molecules, producing two net ATP molecules and two NADH molecules. This is the first step in cellular respiration. [**Section 5.3**]

glycosidic linkage
The bond holding two monosaccharides together. [**Section 5.1**]

guanine
One of the four aromatic bases found in DNA and RNA. Guanine is a purine; it pairs with cytosine. [**Section 7.2**]

heterochromatin
Densely packed, tightly coiled DNA that is generally inactive (not being transcribed). [**Section 7.2**]

hexokinase
The enzyme that catalyzes the phosphorylation of glucose to form glucose-6-phosphate in the first step of glycolysis. This is one of the main regulatory steps of this pathway. Hexokinase is feedback-inhibited by glucose-6-P. [**Section 5.3**]

histones
Globular proteins that assist in DNA packaging in eukaryotes. Histones form octamers around which DNA is wound to form a nucleosome. [**Section 7.2**]

hydrolase
A generic term for an enzyme that hydrolyzes chemical bonds (ATPases, proteases, etc.). [**Section 4.4**]

induced fit model
This model of enzyme-substrate interaction asserts that the active site and the substrate differ slightly in structure/shape and that binding of the substrate induces a conformational change in the enzyme. [**Section 4.5**]

insulin
A peptide hormone produced and secreted by the β-cells of the pancreas. Insulin targets all cells in the body, especially the liver and muscle, and allows them to take glucose out of the blood (thus lowering blood glucose levels). [**Section 5.5**]

isoelectric point
The pH at which an amino acid has no overall charge. [**Section 4.2**]

isomerase
An enzyme that rearranges bonds within a molecule. [**Section 4.4**]

ketogenesis
The production of ketone bodies from fats and protein during times of starvation; it occurs in the liver. [**Section 6.6**]

ketone bodies
Produced from acetyl-CoA under starvation conditions. Ketone bodies can cross the blood brain barrier to act as a fuel source for the brain. [**Section 6.6**]

kinase
An enzyme that transfers a phosphoryl group from ATP to other compounds. Kinases are frequently used in regulatory pathways, phosphorylating other enzymes. [**Sections 4.4 and 4.6**]

K_a
The acid-dissociation constant. The larger the K_a value, the stronger the acid. [**Section 3.4**]

K_b
The base-dissociation constant. The larger the K_b value, the stronger the base. [**Section 3.4**]

K_m
The substrate concentration required to reach $1/2\ V_{max}$; a measure of an enzyme's affinity for its substrate. [**Section 4.7**]

Krebs cycle
The third stage of cellular respiration, in which acetyl-CoA is combined with oxaloacetate to form citric acid. The citric acid is then decarboxylated twice and isomerized to recreate oxaloacetate. In the process, 3 molecules of NADH, 1 molecule of $FADH_2$, and 1 molecule of GTP are formed. [**Section 5.3**]

lactic acid
Produced in muscle cells from the reduction of pyruvate (under anaerobic conditions) to regenerate NAD^+ so that glycolysis can continue. A rise in lactic acid levels usually accompanies an increase in physical activity. [**Section 3.4**]

Le Châtelier's Principle
A principle that describes the effect of changes in the temperature, pressure, or concentration of one of the reactants or products of a reaction at equilibrium. It states that when a system at equilibrium is subjected to a stress, it will shift in the direction that minimizes the effect of this stress. [**Section 3.1**]

Lewis acid/base
Lewis acids are electron-pair acceptors; Lewis bases are electron-pair donors. [**Section 3.4**]

lipoproteins
Large conglomerations of protein, fats, and cholesterol that transport lipids in the bloodstream. [**Section 6.4**]

lipid
A hydrophobic molecule, usually formed from long hydrocarbon chains. The most common forms in which lipids are found in the body are as triglycerides (energy storage), phospholipids (cell membranes), and cholesterol (cell membranes and steroid synthesis). [**Section 6.1**]

lyase
An enzyme that breaks chemical bonds by means other than oxidation or hydrolysis (e.g., pyruvate decarboxylase). [**Section 4.4**]

matrix
The interior of a mitochondrion (the region bounded by the inner membrane). The matrix is the site of action of the pyruvate dehydrogenase complex and the Krebs cycle. [**Section 5.3**]

mitochondrion
An organelle surrounded by a double-membrane (two lipid bilayers) where ATP production takes place. The interior (matrix) is where PDC and the Krebs cycle occur, and the inner membrane contains the enzymes of the electron transport chain and ATP synthase. [**Section 5.3**]

mixed-type inhibition
An enzyme inhibitor that can bind to the enzyme either in its free form or as enzyme-substrate complex. [**Section 4.8**]

NADH
The reduced form (carries electrons) of NAD^+ (nicotinamide adenine dinucleotide). This is the most common electron carrier in cellular respiration. [**Section 5.3**]

negative feedback
See "feedback inhibition." [Section 4.6]

non-coding RNA
RNA that is not translated into protein, includes tRNA and rRNA (both involved in protein synthesis), and snRNA, miRNA, and siNRA (that help regulate gene expression). [Section 7.3]

noncompetitive inhibitor
An enzyme inhibitor that binds at a site other than the active site of an enzyme (i.e., binds at an *allosteric site*). This changes the three-dimensional shape of the enzyme such that it can no longer catalyze the reaction. [Section 4.8]

nucleoside
A structure composed of a ribose molecule linked to one of the aromatic bases. In a deoxynucleoside, the ribose is replaced with deoxyribose. [Section 7.2]

nucleosome
A structure composed of two coils of DNA wrapped around an octet of histone proteins. The nucleosome is the primary form of packaging of eukaryotic DNA. [Section 7.2]

nucleotide
A nucleoside with one or more phosphate groups attached. Nucleoside triphosphates (NTPs) are the building blocks of RNA and are also used as energy molecules, especially ATP. Deoxynucleoside triphosphates (dNTPs) are the building blocks of DNA; in these molecules, the ribose is replaced with deoxyribose. [Section 7.2]

oxaloacetate
A four-carbon molecule that binds with the two-carbon acetyl unit of acetyl-CoA to form citric acid in the first step of the Krebs cycle. [Section 5.3]

oxidation
A process that attaches oxygen, removes hydrogen, or removes electrons from a molecule. [Section 3.3]

oxidative phosphorylation
The oxidation of high-energy electron carriers (NADH and $FADH_2$) coupled to the phosphorylation of ADP, producing ATP. In eukaryotes, oxidative phosphorylation occurs in the mitochondria. [Section 5.3]

oxidoreductase
A class of enzymes that runs redox reactions; this class includes oxidases, reductases, dehydrogenases, etc. [Section 4.4]

pentose phosphate pathway (PPP)
A metabolic pathway that diverts glucose-6-P from glycolysis in order to form ribose-5-P, which can be used to synthesize nucleotides. It also produces NADPH, which can be used as reducing power in fatty acid synthesis. [Section 5.7]

PEPCK
Phosphoenolpyruvate carboxykinase; decarboxylates and phosphorylates oxaloacetate to form phosphoenolpyruvate in the second step of gluconeogenesis. [Section 5.4]

pH
The negative log of [H^+]; the lower the pH the more acidic the solution. [Section 3.4]

phosphatase
An enzyme that dephosphorylates (or removes a phosphoryl group) from a compound. [Section 4.4]

phosphofructokinase (PFK)
The enzyme that catalyzes the phosphorylation of fructose-6-phosphate to form fructose-1-6-bisphosphate in the third step of glycolysis. This is the main regulatory step of glycolysis. PFK is feedback-inhibited by ATP. [Section 5.3]

phospholipid
The primary membrane lipid. Phospholipids consist of a glycerol molecule esterified to two fatty acid chains and a phosphate molecule. Additional, highly hydrophilic groups are attached to the phosphate, making this molecule extremely amphipathic. [Section 6.3]

phosphorylase
An enzyme that transfers a free-floating inorganic phosphate to another molecule. [Section 4.4]

pK_a
The negative log of the K_a value. The lower the pK_a, the stronger the acid. [Section 3.4]

pK_b
The negative log of the K_b value. The lower the pK_b, the stronger the base. [Section 3.4]

pOH
The negative log of [OH^-]; the lower the pOH, the more basic the solution. [Section 3.4]

polyprotic acid
An acid with more than one ionizable proton. [Section 3.4]

polysaccharides
Multiple monosaccharides joined in a large polymer. Polysaccharides are often storage molecules for glucose (glycogen, starch) or structural molecules (cellulose). [Section 5.2]

primary structure
The amino acid sequence of a protein. [**Section 4.3**]

prostaglandins
Eicosanoids derived from 20-carbon fatty acids, prostaglandins have different roles in different tissues, such as regulating smooth muscle contraction, increasing mucus secretion, regulating blood vessel diameter, etc. [**Section 6.5**]

prosthetic group
A non-protein, but organic, molecule (such as a vitamin) that is covalently bound to an enzyme as part of the active site. [**Section 5.3**]

protease
A class of enzymes that hydrolyzes peptide bonds (e.g., trypsin and pepsin). [**Section 4.3**]

purine bases
Aromatic bases found in DNA and RNA that are derived from purine. They have a double-ring structure and include adenine and guanine. [**Section 7.1**]

pyrimidine bases
Aromatic bases found in DNA and RNA that have a single-ring structure. They include cytosine, thymine, and uracil. [**Section 7.1**]

pyruvate dehydrogenase complex
A group of three enzymes that decarboxylates pyruvate, creating an acetyl group and carbon dioxide. The acetyl group is then attached to coenzyme A to produce acetyl-CoA, a substrate in the Krebs cycle. In the process, NAD^+ is reduced to NADH. The pyruvate dehydrogenase complex is the second stage of cellular respiration. [**Section 5.3**]

pyruvate carboxylase
An enzyme that adds CO_2 to pyruvate to form oxaloacetate in the first step of gluconeogenesis. [**Section 5.4**]

pyruvate kinase
An enzyme that catalyzes the final step in glycolysis, the conversion of PEP into pyruvate. [**Section 5.3**]

pyruvic acid
The product of glycolysis; 2 pyruvic acid (pyruvate) molecules are produced from a single glucose molecule. In the absence of oxygen, pyruvic acid undergoes fermentation and is reduced to either lactic acid or ethanol; in the presence of oxygen, pyruvic acid is oxidized to produce acetyl-CoA, which can enter the Krebs cycle. [**Section 5.3**]

quaternary structure
A level of protein structure that involves interactions between side chains of amino acids in separate peptides of a multisubunit protein. [**Section 4.4**]

reaction coupling
Using the energy released by a spontaneous reaction to drive a non-spontaneous reaction; the most often coupled reaction is ATP hydrolysis. [**Section 4.4**]

reciprocal control
The tight regulatory control exerted over opposing metabolic pathways in order to avoid futile cycling. [**Section 5.5**]

reduction
A process that removes oxygen, adds hydrogen, or adds electrons to a molecule. [**Section 3.3**]

replication
The duplication of DNA. [**Section 7.2**]

secondary structure
Hydrogen bonding between the backbone atoms of amino acids in a protein; includes alpha helices and beta pleated sheets. [**Section 4.3**]

sphingolipid
A molecule similar to a phospholipid, except that the backbone is sphingosine instead of glycerol. [**Section 6.5**]

substrate(s)
The reactants in an enzyme-catalyzed reaction. Substrate binds at the active site of an enzyme. [**Section 4.5**]

telomere
A specialized region at the ends of eukaryotic chromosomes that contains several repeats of a particular DNA sequence. These ends are maintained (in some cells) with the help of a special DNA polymerase called *telomerase*. In cells that lack telomerase, the telomeres slowly degrade with each round of DNA replication; this is thought to contribute to the eventual death of the cell. [**Section 7.2**]

terpenes
A member of a broad class of compounds built from isoprene units (C_5H_8). [**Section 6.4**]

tertiary structure
A level of protein structure that involves side chain interactions between amino acids in a protein; produces the three-dimensional shape of the protein. [**Section 4.3**]

thymine
One of the four aromatic bases found in DNA. Thymine is a pyrimidine; it pairs with adenine. [**Section 7.2**]

transcription
The enzymatic process of reading a strand of DNA to produce a complementary strand of RNA. [**Section 6.6**]

transition state (TS)
A high-energy, temporary compound produced during a chemical reaction. The energy required to produce TS (the activation energy) determines the rate of the reaction. [**Section 3.2**]

translation
The process of reading a strand of mRNA to synthesize protein. Protein translation takes place on a ribosome. [**Section 7.3**]

tricarboxylic acid (TCA) cycle
See "Krebs cycle." [**Section 5.3**]

triglyceride
Three fatty acids bound to a glycerol molecule. This is an energy storage molecule for the body. [**Section 6.2**]

uncompetitive inhibition
An enzyme inhibitor that can bind to the enzyme only after its substrate has bound. Uncompetitive inhibitors appear to increase the affinity an enzyme has for its substrate because it effectively locks the two together. [**Section 4.8**]

uracil
One of four aromatic bases found in RNA. Uracil is pyrimidine; it pairs with adenine. [**Section 7.3**]

waxes
Long-chain fats esterified to long-chain alcohols. Waxes form waterproof barriers. [**Section 6.5**]